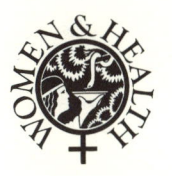

Women and Health
*Cultural and Social
Perspectives*

Women in Labor

Mothers, Medicine, and Occupational Health in the United States, 1890–1980

Allison L. Hepler

Ohio State University Press / *Columbus*

All photographs and illustrations, except as indicated, are courtesy of the National Archives and Records Administration, College Park, Maryland.

Copyright © 2000 by The Ohio State University.
All rights reserved.

Library of Congress Cataloging-in-Publication Data

Hepler, Allison L.
  Women in labor : mothers, medicine, and occupational health in the United States, 1890–1980 / Allison L. Hepler.
    p. cm.—(Women and health)
  Includes bibliographical references and index.
    ISBN 0-8142-0850-9 — ISBN 0-8142-5055-6 (alk. paper)
    1. Women—Employment—Health aspects—United States—History. 2. Industrial hygiene—United States—History. I. Title. II. Women & health (Columbus, Ohio)
    RC963.6.W65 H47 2000
    616.98′03′082—dc21
                        00-008776

Text design by Mira Nenonen.
Cover design by Diane Gleba Hall.
Type set in Adobe Garamond by Graphic Composition, Inc.
Printed by Thomson-Shore, Inc.

The paper used in this publication meets the minimum requirements of the American National Standard for Information Sciences—Permanence of Paper for Printed Library Materials. ANSI Z39.48-1992.

9 8 7 6 5 4 3 2 1

To Bob's memory
. . . it carries me far indeed.

Contents

Series Editors' Foreword	ix
Acknowledgments	xi
Introduction	1
1 The Effects of Double Duty	11
2 Industrial Poisons: *The Two-Percent Solution*	28
3 Industrial Health in an Industrializing World	46
4 Women in Wartime Industries: *"We Want Steel Toes like the Men"*	67
5 Alice Hamilton and the Equal Rights Amendment	83
6 Women and the Environment: *"The Pathology and Hygiene of Housework"*	102
7 Factories, Feminism, and Fetal Protection Policies	113
Epilogue	127
List of Abbreviations	131
Notes	133
Bibliography	161
Index	171

Series Editors' Foreword

Allison Hepler's history of women and occupational health in the United States offers a richly detailed examination of a crucial historical subject that is, as well, a significant contemporary issue. Women's labor force participation rates are expected to grow in the twenty-first century. The workplace hazards that threaten women in this new century will clearly be different than those encountered in previous generations, but many of the issues to be settled and questions to be answered will remain the same. How will problems be uncovered and scientific evidence amassed about them? Through what political negotiations and under what economic circumstances will these problems be controlled? How will society mediate between understandings of women's health that stress women's differences from men—particularly in the area of reproduction—and those understandings that rest upon the similarities of threats facing all of those employed in particular occupations? How will women's increasing participation in the military and their battlefield exposures change perceptions of occupational health? *Women in Labor,* with its historical perspective, is enlightening and vital to understanding the complexities of the issues we will be confronting. We are pleased to include this valuable and critical study in the Women and Health series of the Ohio State University Press.

Acknowledgments

It is hard to believe that I began this book six years ago. The intellectual and literary talents I have acquired during this period have come from a variety of sources. Morris J. Vogel's good-natured patience, fine-tuned criticism, and creativity turned an enthusiastic if somewhat unfocused graduate student into a historian. Margaret Marsh and Allen Davis, the other members of my dissertation committee at Temple University, deserve equally high praise. Professor Marsh's encouragement and key remarks at critical stages of this research have especially sharpened my own instincts in analyzing sources. Professor Davis's expertise in reformers and reform helped me think beyond the boundaries of this work.

Historians elsewhere, especially those attending the American Association for the History of Medicine conferences and the Berkshire Conferences on the History of Women, have likewise provided wonderful intellectual challenges. I am particularly grateful to David Rosner, whose generous advice and comments in the early stages of my work were a great source of encouragement. I am also thankful for the feedback and support I received from Rima Apple, Patricia Evridge Hill, the late Jack Pressman, Lynne Page Snyder, Judith Walzer Leavitt, Jill Cooper, Patricia Reeve, Claudia Clark, Elizabeth Toon, Jennifer Gunn, and Carolyn Malone.

To my colleagues at the Maine Women's Studies Consortium, the various University of Maine campuses, and especially the University of Maine at Farmington, I offer my appreciation for their curiosity and insights. Seth Wigderson, Mazie Hough, Carol Toner, Eileen Eagan, Diana Long, Lee Sharkey, Norma Johnsen, and Cathleen McAnneny have been and continue to be enormously helpful. The interdisciplinary approach characteristic of UMF has greatly broadened my understanding of the many issues and perspectives associated with motherhood and medicine. Students in history and in women's studies at UMF have continued to help teach me how to ground my academic interests.

The Temple University community, while I was a graduate student and later, kept me focused on both the small picture and that picture's larger significance; I benefited greatly from my association with Sally Dwyer-McNulty, Susan Morse, Julie Berebitsky, John Kokolus, Christie Balka, and Mary Pileggi.

UMF's Faculty Development Committee and especially the Department of Social Sciences and Business have provided funding for attendance at conferences, clerical help, and enormous technical and moral support. Some of my research was supported by grants: one such grant came from the Medical College of Pennsylvania's Archives and Special Collections on Women in Medicine, and another from the American College of Obstetricians and Gynecologists—Ortho Fellowship in the History of Medicine. Parts of this book have appeared in other publications, and I am grateful to the publishers for permission to reprint those portions. "'And We Want Steel Toes Like the Men': Gender and Occupational Health during World War II" appeared in the Winter 1998 issue of the *Bulletin of the History of Medicine;* "'Shaping the Life of the Pre-Natal': Labor Laws, Liability and Lead Poisoning of Women in Industry in Twentieth-Century United States" appeared in the Spring 1999 issue of *Social Politics.*

I was fortunate to have clear and direct help of all sorts from the staff of Ohio State University Press. I learned more than I like to admit from Ruth Melville and Nancy Woodington. Although Janet Golden's early support and sound editorial advice in the later stages of this manuscript helped me sharpen my arguments, I alone am responsible for the final product.

My thanks also go to friends and family who have shared their homes with me while I conducted my research. I am particularly grateful to Jocelyn Douglass and to all the Homan family, whose hospitality I counted on more times than I can recall. An amazing assortment of friends and family members showed great patience in at least accepting the single-mindedness of this pursuit, even if they did not always ask too many questions about it. One exception is Mary Homan, whose experience as a mother and a teacher led to many helpful, wide-ranging conversations about the balance between home and work. Another is Rob Stevens; his humor and curiosity made me answer some interesting and hard questions about work.

While the dissertation and this book might have been written without help from some of those already mentioned, it could not have been written without Bob Miller, who was my husband and my best friend. To make the move to graduate school possible, he agreed to sell the dream house we had built. To help me out of the balancing act that making money and making time for research and writing imposes, he worked two jobs. When I had to struggle to describe this endeavor as worthwhile, he believed in me and defended what to many seemed like an uncertain venture. Bob, a woodworker, photographer, and writer, died in a work accident three months before I received a contract from Ohio State University Press to write this book. I am very proud of what we accomplished together, and I view this book as a very small, but I hope worthy, part of that legacy.

Introduction

Regardless of what our own workplace environment looks like, occupational health touches nearly every part of our lives—not only in the taxes we pay to support state and federal labor laws but also in the quality of the clothes we wear and of the food we eat. Those of us unfortunate enough to work in unhealthy environments may experience occupational health issues more intimately—in headaches, respiratory problems, backaches and other muscular injuries, skin rashes, and any number of "silent" hazards with long latency periods.

Ideas about occupational health are not created in a vacuum. They are the complex product of political, economic, social, and cultural pressures by employers, workers, state and federal health officials, and physicians. Often they lie beyond the traditional confines of management-labor negotiation. For instance, an employer, at the insistence of other manufacturers, decides that installing blowers to dissipate hazardous fumes is too costly and that respirators for workers in the plant will provide adequate protection. The workers, especially those who wear glasses, view respirators as a nuisance, and some of them decide not to wear them. They prefer the blowers. Public health officials prepare statistics that show smoking as a greater health risk to workers than what they breathe at work. Elected officials in the state want to keep this plant from relocating overseas because of the high costs of complying with health regulations. Each has a stake in what defines a healthy workplace, and medical science is never the only factor.

Gender is only beginning to be considered as a significant factor in understanding what it has meant to be healthy on the job. Gender is best defined as the social roles that prescribe what it means to be male and female. These roles are shaped partly by biology, but perhaps more by an educational system that coerces boys into certain careers, media that characterize the ideal female figure, and family behavior that can sometimes reinforce, or defy, stereotypes. The inclusion of gender complicates the picture of occupational health; including the experiences of women in the workplace requires a redefinition of "workplace." It is also necessary to consider how women's capacity to be mothers—and the accompanying social expectation that women raise children—resulted in different definitions of workplace health for women and for men.

A number of critical questions arise in examining questions of gender and workplace health. How has protective labor legislation influenced women's lives and men's lives, both in and out of the workplace? How did employers, reformers, and medical professionals determine which jobs were too dangerous for women, and to what extent did fears about motherhood influence those decisions? How did occupational health laws reflect prevailing gender norms? How have changes in the practice of medicine affected gender norms? How did the debate over the Equal Rights Amendment shape the workplace? To what extent have occupational safety and health concerns, particularly those related to women, been socially constructed?

In answering these questions, one must look at how ideas about motherhood and womanhood changed during the twentieth century. In many ways, workplace conditions shaped women's social identity. Laws that limited women's hours of work both reflected and reinforced a definition of motherhood that implied the primacy of household and child-rearing duties, a recognition and an acceptance that wage-earning women did indeed perform a double duty. Attention paid to women workers' health required an understanding of their home life, while male workers faced no such expectation.

Employers' attention to biological hazards in the workplace by midcentury, as evidenced by the implementation of fetal protection policies, suggests a narrower view of "mothering." Rules that forbade a woman to handle chemicals that adversely affected her reproductive system emphasized her childbearing role over her child-rearing one. Responsibility for workplace health shifted from the state to the employer and ultimately to the individual. Health promoters focused on personal habits—washing hands, for example—more than on environmental efforts. While this narrower focus can arguably be viewed as advancing women's opportunities and recognizing the variety of women's roles, because social roles did not change as much as economic roles did, this often meant that women were expected to "do it all." Without the protection from overwork promised by labor laws directed at females, the "double day" became the norm for millions of women.

This book examines the experiences of wage-earning women and men in twentieth-century United States against the backdrop of changes in medicine, the political landscape, the industrial environment, and the workforce. All of these changes reveal ways in which gender norms helped construct concepts of occupational health and disease. Employment policies represented common societal notions about motherhood as they evolved in the twentieth century. Also, changing ideas about motherhood mirrored changes in medicine that increasingly reflected a narrower understanding of disease. And it is impossible to understand employment policies for both men and women without examining the influences of the various feminist ideologies that waxed and waned in this century, producing contradictory results for workers.

The worldview of Progressive Era reformers interested in the welfare of working-class women was dominated by a broad understanding of motherhood. These "maternalists," according to Linda Gordon, viewed a woman's primary responsibility in society as motherhood, and their definition of "mother" went well beyond just "childbearing female." Reformers characterized motherhood broadly; a mother's duties also included caring for and rearing children and maintaining a safe, moral, and healthful household environment. In this view, "hazard" was also defined broadly. Many women in this era could not be full-time mothers because they had to work for wages. Employment policies regarding women's health and safety in the factory, therefore, tried to accommodate this reality—limiting the hours that women could work in the workplace and prohibiting them from working nights, which presumably kept working mothers from overexposure to industrial hazards and from being too fatigued to perform their household duties. In the twentieth century these policies became more specific and more tightly organized around women's biological capabilities as mothers. What was considered hazardous also became limited to specific chemicals in the workplace. But gender differences, however defined, were used both to promote and to hinder women's advancement in society and in the workplace.[1] This book's emphasis on the relationship between motherhood, the workplace, and health demonstrates how private concerns about children become subjects of public policy and debate at certain historical moments. While historians interested in motherhood have explored issues of maternal and infant health, less attention has been paid to the exclusion of women from jobs that exposed them to reproductive dangers.[2]

Changes in medical practice promoted an ever narrower view of what was considered hazardous to successful motherhood. New medical ideas also helped redefine public and private health concerns. At the beginning of the century, "scientific medicine," with its emphasis on the specific pathogen and the individual cell, had reoriented many medical professionals and practitioners away from medicine's older, more holistic view of the patient within his or her environment. The actions of reformers interested in workplace health, and especially women's health, show, however, that the older attitudes toward health and disease still held considerable sway. Reformers believed that causes of illness were not limited to what could be seen under a microscope. Historians of medicine have appreciated the role of medical authority in influencing women's lives, particularly with respect to reproduction, but many aspects of modern medicine are not as easily understood when applied to the experiences of working women. When one considers health in the workplace, where "women's work" more easily traversed the boundaries between home and workplace, it becomes very clear that modern medicine is not as specialized as many have thought. As long as the wage-earning mother also continues to be the primary caregiver and housekeeper, historians must consider how physicians and public health officials bent the dictates of modern medicine to fit the more complicated reality of the workplace. Analyzing the interaction between old and new theories about medicine with respect to women's lives removes the subject of motherhood from a dichotomous public-private framework, making it more complicated.[3]

In addition to looking at workplace issues, this book extends the traditional limits of environmental history. Work in this field, begun out of moral concern for the planet, has recently been shaped by endemic, structural issues of more long-term and global significance.[4] Historians have begun to view gender as a crucial component of good environmental history, especially with respect to biological and social reproduction. I wish to remind readers not only of the variety of definitions of "environmentalism" that antedated the 1960s but also of the variety of gender influences that have influenced recent events.[5] For instance, we can reconcile Lois Gibbs's "motherly instincts," which led to the Love Canal revelations in the 1970s, with widespread opposition to fetal protection policies by women in industry during the same period—if we understand how women, in their capacity as mothers, have historically related to their environment, and how, in their capacity as workers, they have increasingly sought the right to define motherhood for themselves.[6]

Threats to motherhood carried political implications, especially with respect to how women were "protected." Historians of protective labor legislation, who have tended to focus on the impact of hours restrictions, as well as on assumptions about working women's "morality," have noted that many agendas were operating, only some of which actually protected motherhood. For example, reformers concerned with the health of mothers and future mothers admitted that protection sometimes meant sex or class discrimination. For industry, economic imperatives shaped protection, which meant that employers sometimes ignored known risks to motherhood because they could hire women at lower wages than men. In turn, male workers and their unions, who sometimes found their jobs jeopardized by women's employment, tried to safeguard their own positions by "protecting" women out of certain jobs. The state, which believed it had a mandate to protect women and children, had to balance a variety of considerations; it found it could not effectively protect all women from occupational hazards, especially those found in such traditionally low-paying female jobs as domestic service, agriculture, and nonprofessional nursing. Some agendas supported excluding women from workplaces where there were known reproductive hazards.[7]

Finally, the politics of feminism inform this research because of the long-standing tensions among those called feminists. The existence of working women's double duty led many feminist reformers in the first half of this century to support laws and policies that limited the number of hours women could work in the workplace. These reformers understood that women's social responsibilities differed from men's. Other feminists, however, believed that such regulations institutionalized women's inequality in the workplace, and that only by letting women compete with men on equal (i.e., men's) terms would gender equality prevail. The distinction between difference and equality still informs feminist positions on women's status in the workplace. Recent court decisions, seen by some feminists as victories in the war on sex discrimination, have been viewed by others as generating only an equal right to a hazardous workplace. Accepting one position over another had and still has its pitfalls. Ignoring women's biological differences from men runs the risk of de-emphasizing the significance of the act of childbearing. Emphasizing similarities to men risks defining women by male norms. Accentuating gender differences, however, tends to separate men and women artificially, stressing social characteristics over individual talents.

Understanding the important and long-lasting relationship between feminism and occupational health sheds light on contemporary debates over the significance of sex and difference. The Equal Rights Amendment debate in the 1920s centered on the protective and discriminatory aspects of protective labor legislation. While many historians have noted the institutionalization of protectionist policies at the state and federal levels in the 1920s, the impact of pro-ERA feminists on occupational health has not received as much scholarly attention. Historians of feminism have only recently begun to focus on the similar goals of different groups of feminists. My research documents the extent to which various feminisms influenced the direction of workplace health. A close examination of the rhetoric surrounding working women's health supports arguments that twentieth-century feminism represented a complex intersection of new and old constructions of gender equality and difference derived from scientific, social, political, and cultural forces.[8]

This lingering interaction between science and feminism is best represented by examining the long career of Alice Hamilton, an internationally known toxicologist. A longtime supporter of protective labor legislation, Hamilton changed her mind about the Equal Rights Amendment in 1952, at the age of eighty-three. I believe that Hamilton's attention to workplace health for nearly half a century gave her the opportunity to keep the worker foremost in her mind while remaining aware of the multitude of interests that did not share her priorities. A physician and an alumna of Hull House, she balanced her scientific training with her social concerns, adjusting both but never emphasizing the former to the neglect of the latter. Her actions as a protectionist feminist offer valuable insight into the ways she balanced social norms and individual differences, and how she continued to respond to social and economic changes throughout her life. She became an equal-rights feminist only after changes in both the workplace and the status of women had persuaded her that categorical distinctions between men and women had become less significant than individual distinctions. Only after environmental conditions (both material and social) had changed sufficiently did she feel comfortable relinquishing state responsibility for working women's health in favor of more individual relationships between worker and employer.[9]

The analysis of gender norms is pivotal to this book's most significant claims, but other analyses should also be mentioned. Those concerned with women's reproductive health in the workplace were, for the most part, white and middle class. Most of their research focused on white, working-class women. On their survey forms, Women's Bureau researchers often noted subjects' racial and ethnic backgrounds. Occasionally they focused their research on African-American women in specific industries, but the sources reveal little with respect to race or racial agendas. The patterns established by gender stereotypes, however, are instructive. As employers began to consider gender in terms of physiological difference, they also began to look at racial and ethnic traits more narrowly in employment decisions.

Historians have viewed protective labor legislation as a method for one class to enforce its norms on another. Middle-class women insisting that working-class women share the same values, values that favor full-time motherhood over earning power, seems class-based, but it has always been more complex than that. Many proponents of gender-based protective legislation also supported increases in women's wages, and it seems clear that some working-class women did share some middle-class women's values but lacked the means to achieve them. The 1991 *United Automobile Workers v. Johnson Controls, Inc.* case is also instructive here. When the U.S. Supreme Court decided that an employer could not legally prohibit women from working in areas of high lead concentration, Johnson Controls closed its doors and moved out of the country. It believed that the costs of changing the workplace were prohibitive in the United States. While viewed as a victory by many middle-class feminists, the decision effectively deprived Bennington, Vermont, of one of its best-paying blue-collar workplaces for both women and men. But it was not middle-class women who had brought the lawsuit. It was the women workers themselves.[10] Then, as now, class identity is complicated by other forms of consciousness.

This story begins in the late nineteenth century, when attention to occupational health was rooted in an understanding of working people's material conditions. This view also supported a woman's primary role as that of mother and housewife, even if she worked for wages outside the home. As a result, factory reformers saw a highly gendered world where the workplace environment deeply affected the home. Reformers believed that changing this environment would improve an entire society at risk from any number of dangerous industrial conditions. They promoted a number of sanitary reforms and a variety of industrial welfare measures, the most long-lasting of which resulted in gender-specific protective labor laws. These laws, aimed at ensuring the maternal health of all women, primarily restricted the number of hours women could work for wages. Despite this environmentalist perspective, modern science had begun to influence the workplace, most notably in studies done on fatigue as a physiological condition, and in such cases as *Muller v. Oregon*. Both the studies and *Muller* gave scientific sanction to broadly applied protective labor laws.

Adopting modern medicine's emphasis on the specific, a few reformers also began to express concerns about physiological risks that the workplace posed to motherhood, especially with the expanded use of chemical poisons like lead and benzene. In some cases state policies regulating the workplace resulted, but most research and activism in the area of poisons took place outside governmental structures. Consequently, despite the attention to the biological aspects of motherhood, most official advocacy during this period revolved around its social aspects.

By the 1920s, a variety of modern medical practices had become institutionalized in various state and federal agencies concerned with workers' health and with women in industry, creating yet another relationship between occupational and non-occupational health. The introduction of an Equal Rights Amendment in Congress affected employment policies primarily because of the amendment's potential impact on protective labor legislation. Despite the presence of many anti-ERA protectionists in policymaking positions, ERA supporters also shaped workplace health practices. Urging the use of individual rather than gender characteristics in determining job suitability helped employers in their efforts to shift responsibility for workplace health to the individual worker.

Protectionism, ironically, produced the same result. Protectionist efforts in the 1920s and 1930s to identify and understand the relationships between home, workplace, and health had the unintended consequence of providing support for employers' attempts to identify a worker's personal behavior—rather than conditions in the workplace—as the primary cause of ill health on the job. Both approaches served to reduce attention to environmental causes of industrial disease.

World War II forced employers and women workers into a new accommodation between home and workplace, but only after first implementing policies that de-emphasized gender differences and instead targeted individual qualifications. The federal government also downplayed the hazards of the industrial workplace, legitimizing the "equal treatment" philosophy and reinforcing employer policies that supported individual responsibility for health. Eventually, however, women workers forced employers and the government to recognize that female health, at least as measured by high absenteeism rates, required special considerations. This dual treatment of women workers advanced women's equal opportunities in the workplace and at the same time caused a recognition of the different social responsibilities of men and women workers. As a society, we are still trying to do both without sacrificing either.

Wartime experiences sparked a postwar revival of interest in passing an Equal Rights Amendment, and since much of this book examines the construction of "difference" among women and between women and men, an analysis of debates over the ERA reveals some interesting insights. Society moved away from a public health–oriented campaign undertaken on behalf of all women, whose primary social roles involved the household and motherhood, and toward a more complex and diverse view of women. Women's livelihoods seemed better protected by employment policies that considered workers' individual suitability for certain jobs. In many ways, these two positions resembled two different theories about health. The evolution of modern medicine helped shape occupational health policies for women as these policies became more clearly defined by physiology than by social roles.

In many ways workplace conditions had improved for both men and women by the 1950s, setting the stage for more substantive shifts in gender roles at work and in society by the 1960s and 1970s. As early as 1952, protective labor laws began to be challenged, and governmental interest in occupational health declined. Employers, however, began to institute "fetal protection policies," ostensibly based on scientific evidence but also reflective of legal changes that increased economic uncertainty in predicting business insurance costs. By the late 1940s, courts had begun to pay more attention to the rights of children damaged in utero.

While some aspects of occupational health similarly became more narrowly defined, growing public concerns about environmental hazards in the 1960s initiated a widespread consumer-based movement. The movement gave rise to complex ties between the public environment and the more private environments of the workplace and of the household. In some ways this brings us full circle from the early years of the century.

Several things remained constant throughout the twentieth century. First, gender roles, especially those associated with motherhood, influenced workplace health policies for men and women. These policies increasingly recognized the variety of women's roles. Medical theories of disease, economic imperatives of doing business, and a variety of feminisms influenced both gender roles and workplace policies. And the tensions within both medicine and feminism both improved and threatened the health of all workers at different times. These various relationships weave the story together.

Historical dilemmas endure. Women are treated as equals in the workplace but without equivalent wages or help with housework. They are glorified as mothers of the next generation but lack the economic independence to fill their roles properly. They can be acknowledged as biological mothers, but their fetuses may be seen as more important than themselves. They are sometimes viewed as individuals with unique talents but at other times losing their identity by implicitly accepting workplace rules designed for males.

Today, with a relatively well-developed legal construct of fetal personhood, some argue that women have been reduced to vessels for children. This is an odd and discomfiting construction of motherhood. At the turn of the last century society also deemed women's role as mothers valuable, but it defined motherhood differently. The combined influences of gender, medical theories of disease, feminism, and economic priorities shaped, perhaps altered that definition.

1
The Effects of Double Duty

In 1894 Robert Watchorn, the chief factory inspector of Pennsylvania, urged an audience of his peers to pay attention to the hidden "hundreds of untimely deaths" of working people caused by insufficient regard for ventilation and sanitation in the workplace. He criticized industry's "pitiful and miserable efforts" to reduce its highly visible industrial accidents when "a defective sanitary system, together with an insufficient supply of ventilation, has slain . . . tens of thousands [of workers]." Watchorn described the big killer's silent and effective route: "[It] steals his victims by a slower but not less sure method, creeping into their vitals, and making its citadel there, pours out its insidious poisons, not only to the destruction of the life of such victims but all too frequently entailing on society a race of consumptives and weaklings, who often become paupers and a menace to public health."[1]

Watchorn explained the specific mixture of elements that made poor ventilation so deadly. It was not the mere lack of air, he said, but the impregnation of the "already vitiated atmosphere" with "disease and death from the dust and vapors of the chemical works, the cigar factory, the tobacco shop, the bakery, the candy works, the chenille factory, soap works, and worst of all, the room in which old carpets, old clothes contaminated with filth, dirt and disease are torn into shreds for use in the shoddy mills."[2]

Watchorn's plea for better ventilation resonated with his fellow factory inspectors, many of whom had been working in Pennsylvania since the 1892 passage of the state's factory inspection law. They all understood the relationship between the factory environment and disease, having witnessed similar conditions in a variety of industries across the state. They also understood the cause-and-effect relationship between the material conditions of the workplace and unhealthy workers. Finally, although it is hard to tell whether Watchorn and his colleagues actually observed this or were merely speculating, they made the logical connection between workers' bad health and the health of future generations. Watchorn's sentiments imply a very broad view of health, one that involves looking at a person's whole makeup and not only at a specific ailment. His view contradicted medicine's narrower, twentieth-century vision.

Such a narrow view was unacceptable to many with experience in occupational health, and for obvious reasons: the worker's very environment was the cause of many health problems—the fumes breathed, the dust ingested, the chemicals absorbed through the skin. Watchorn and his fellow factory inspectors witnessed this.[3] Wage-earning women were no strangers to this broader view of health; for women who worked outside the home, the workplace environment encompassed a large arena. At the turn of the century women had broad familial responsibilities—childbearing, child-rearing, household duties—which meant that their working hours typically went beyond the time spent earning wages.

Social reformers of the Progressive Era also recognized these blurred boundaries and supported protective labor legislation for women—primarily in the form of shorter hours—to protect working women's abilities to be good mothers in the present and the future. Given the Progressive Era reformers' concerns for children and their fears about race suicide, it made sense for them to privilege women's domestic responsibilities.[4] Their protective labor legislation grew out of an environmentalist worldview—a perspective that recognized broadly defined relationships between health, the environment, and work. Its proponents initially resisted taking a more specialized view of women's health.

To understand modern medicine, we need to understand that the discovery of "germs," as they were called, in the mid-nineteenth century redirected an ancient view of disease, where health had been viewed as the maintenance of balance between bodily intake and outgo as well as the body's relationship to its environment. In this view every part of the human body was connected to every other part. According to Charles Rosenberg, "Equilibrium was synonymous with health, disequilibrium with illness." Bleeding and purging often "cured" disease. Changes in season put people at risk; much sickness (and recovery) occurred during the spring and fall months. The concept of balance also applied to the relationship between physical and moral health. Disease represented a moral failing. Cleanliness represented health; filth caused disease, both physical and mental. A clean environment helped keep people healthy. Since there was an integral relationship among the different parts of the body, physicians had to treat the whole patient, considering the patient's living conditions, diet, and activities.[5]

Translated into public health terms, the "filth theory" of health and disease directed efforts at sanitary reform, especially in urban areas. Historians of medicine have noted the political and economic implications of medical practices, describing nineteenth-century attempts to rid cities of epidemic disease by cleaning up streets and alleys filled with garbage and animal and human excrement. City sewer systems and regular garbage and trash pickups made sense in a world where cholera and yellow fever seemed to affect disproportionately the poorest citizens, who lived in the worst neighborhoods. Such sanitary measures offered tangible relief. While some city and religious leaders believed that illness was caused by the dissolute lifestyle and moral failings of the poor, others noted the cause-and-effect relationship between a bad environment and bad health, trying to eliminate bad health by improving the environment.[6]

Urban environmentalists also witnessed the effects of an unclean environment in the growing number of factories. When young women began to work in the newly built cotton mills in Lowell, Massachusetts, in the 1830s, people soon began to suspect that the mills were breeding grounds for respiratory disease. Cotton dust in the air and the warm, moist, and unventilated quality of that air were believed to cause disease. In addition, as a Lowell physician, John Allen, wrote in 1849, women workers commonly suffered from "varicose veins, dropsical swelling of the feet and limbs, and prolapsus uter [sic]."[7]

Nineteenth-century observers who read Elizabeth Stuart Phelps's novel *The Silent Partner* learned of "cotton-cough" in the textile mills of Massachusetts. According to Phelps's working-class heroine, "It comes from sucking filling through the shuttle." One could readily identify weavers on the street: they were corpse-like women with "bleached yellow faces" and "bright eyes." The factory accommodated the cotton thread, not the workers, according to Phelps, who described hot, humid conditions through the words of her characters: "The temperature has stood at 115° in our room today. It hasn't been below 110° not since last Saturday. It's 125° in the dressing room."[8]

Phelps did not single out women as victims of capitalist greed, nor did early efforts at improving factory conditions focus on female workers. Alice Kessler-Harris has argued that only after the courts struck down a number of laws aimed at regulating male workers' hours and conditions in the 1870s did reformers turn their attention to gender-specific workplace conditions. Their arguments appealed to traditional notions of female weakness and domesticity. After persuading employers and legislators to improve working conditions for women and children, reformers hoped to extend these reforms to all workers.[9]

It is important to examine women's working conditions at the turn of this century in the context of a gendered and environmentalist worldview. When workers, reformers, state labor officials, and even business owners remarked on the relationship between the workplace and the domestic roles of women, they exhibited an environmental understanding of the world not unlike that represented by the filth theory of disease: a world where (1) sickness was caused by something visible, specifically a bad environment; (2) home and workplace were not so easily separated and compartmentalized for working women because they worked in both places (in tenement sweatshops, home and workplace were the same place); and (3) a variety of community and societal roles defined motherhood.[10]

Unhealthy and unsafe industrial conditions attracted the attention of settlement house workers, social welfare reformers, and labor activists, resulting in demands for state action. Factory inspections in Pennsylvania began in 1892 after the passage of laws mandating inspection of industries hiring women and children. Although statistics gathered by the state's factory inspectors meticulously recorded accidents and working conditions by gender as well as by such other categories as age, place of birth, residence, and ethnicity, inspectors interpreted their responsibilities as entailing more than ensuring women's and children's health, safety, and morality. Inspectors were concerned about conditions for all workers, and they used the law as a means of investigating factories. Since the law exempted employers whose total workforce numbered under five, some industries, according to Inspector Isabella Coombs of Pittsburgh, fired women and children or reduced their workforce to avoid inspections.[11]

New Jersey shared its neighbor's concerns about women workers. Its strategy focused more directly on the environmental origins of ill health. Not content to rely solely on rules mandating sex-segregated toilet and washing facilities to raise the general moral tone of plants, New Jersey also introduced mandatory blower regulations in dusty factories employing women and children and called for annual whitewashing and painting to eliminate the accumulation of dust. These measures benefited all employees.[12]

Other industrial states, such as New York, Illinois, and Massachusetts, established factory investigating commissions whose members inspected some of the dirtiest factories. Inspectors were particularly appalled at the working conditions and the health of women and children. To reduce exposure to these conditions, inspectors advocated maximum hours legislation for these "especially susceptible" groups. "In shop and factory and mill all over our country," declared Margaret Dreier Robins, president of the Women's Trade Union League, "women are working under conditions that weaken vitality and sap moral fiber—conditions that are destructive alike to physical health and moral development."[13]

Reformers predicated their concern for women's working conditions on the widespread belief that women's maternal responsibilities—broadly defined to include childbearing, child-rearing, and housekeeping—should be society's first consideration in determining workplace conditions for women. According to James Campbell, Watchorn's successor as Pennsylvania's chief factory inspector in 1897, it was common knowledge that long hours of standing, heat exhaustion, and nervous strain produced "an effect which must tell with power on future generations."[14]

Dr. Mary Putnam Jacobi made the same point in 1896 when she testified before the Reinhard Committee investigating the "Condition of Female Labor" in New York City. She urged the protection of women workers because "the physical health of the women and children is of immense importance—not merely to themselves and family, but to the community at large. It is a social matter, and if the health of thousands and millions of women and children [is] allowed to deteriorate, why the whole nation suffers." In her statement, Jacobi acknowledged that women's workplace conditions affected their home and indeed their community.[15]

Campbell and Jacobi worried most about the effects of overwork on duties at home. Campbell described fatigue caused by specific working conditions. While he could not point to measurable physiological changes in workers, he and others could see the results of long hours, high heat, and the strain caused by constant attention to moving machinery: "pallor, drawn lines of exhaustion about the mouth, nervous, feverish movements," according to one investigator. Long hours of standing or sitting at the factory not only took time away from the care of children, which led to juvenile delinquency, but also made women too tired to perform household tasks properly.[16]

In women who worked nights investigators could see most clearly the effects of double duty. Such women looked tired all the time. A day worker at one New Jersey woolen mill described her counterparts on the night shift: "I see them sometimes in the morning when they come from the mills, their eyes so red, their faces so white, like they come from the grave!" Another was more blunt: "Nightwork kills womans [sic]."[17]

Most married women who worked the night shift did so in order to balance child care with wage earning. Women did housework during the daylight hours after work. Investigators reported that numerous women regularly went from eighteen to twenty-four hours without sleep. A New York State labor investigator talked with a woman who worked nights so she could take care of her "home, garden, cow, and boy." Even if women could find time to sleep during daylight hours, the investigator considered daytime rest "unnatural" and "inferior" because it was "less refreshing and restorative" and almost always "interrupted and less continuous." As a result of these observations and of higher mortality rates among working women, investigators concluded that women were physiologically weaker than men.[18]

Debates over the need to improve these women's health largely took place within the context of women's social roles—their ability to maintain family, household, and community relations. Workers, reformers, and factory inspectors also used statistical and anecdotal evidence to suggest a relationship between factory conditions and female reproductive problems. In Fall River,

Massachusetts, between 1908 and 1912, more women mill workers died from pregnancy- and childbirth-related factors than did non-mill employees.[19] When Campbell warned of the deleterious effects of women's working conditions on future generations, he expressed commonly held beliefs about the declining national birthrate. Standing or sitting for long periods of time, for instance, was said to cause "diseases of the sexual organs," which resulted in miscarriages or sickly children.[20]

Factory reformers' fears about the generational effects of maternal health were informed by turn-of-the-century scientific and social debates about the relative influences of nature and nurture on human evolution. Many reformers supported the Neo-Lamarckian theory that children inherited their parents' acquired characteristics. These environmentally derived traits could result from both positive and negative experiences. Offspring of women factory workers risked inheriting illnesses and debilities caused by dangerous conditions in the workplace. When many World War I draftees exhibited signs of physical and mental unfitness, factory inspectors' and reformers' fears about the social and physical deterioration of the race seemed to have been realized. A Nebraska official had argued in 1907 that "to lower the standard of bodily strength [of women] will bring a disastrous reaction on society later." According to another bureaucrat, too many hours or unhealthy working conditions "injure the mothers of our citizens. . . . Infants are born to die young, or grow into men weak and sickly."[21]

While this theory lost ground as genetic evidence gained favor, it continued to hold sway in the social sciences. Perhaps not surprisingly, many middle-class, college-educated women (and future reformers) gravitated to this position because it offered a means of disproving various scientific theories of female inferiority. At the same time, because this position implicitly acknowledged the relationship between environment and health and tended to reinforce public perceptions of female weakness, it also provided intellectual grounds for gender-based labor laws.[22]

Business owners also recognized the relationship between home and workplace directing their efforts toward making the workplace more homelike. While some of their methods reflect those adopted by advocates of protective labor legislation, many employers had different motives that provide clues to the post–World War I trajectory of occupational health. Business owners were well aware of the effects of environmental health on economic productivity. A Boston Chamber of Commerce survey conducted in 1910 concluded that the common cold accounted for $10,800 in lost wages annually in department stores and manufacturing establishments, among office and medical staff, and, interestingly, housewives. Preventive measures targeted the environment and individuals: "breathe pure air; avoid dust; take regular exercise; get plenty of sleep and rest; . . . and do not sit for long hours in a stuffy, close room."[23]

The chamber's Committee on Prevention of Disease and Accidents, chaired by Dr. James Honeij, distributed informational posters to its members and eventually reached a national audience. Carter's Ink returned the posters, noting the disjunction between the goals of pure air and the reality of the dirty, dusty living conditions of workers. If they were posted, wrote a company representative, "There would be a strong tendency to treat [the issue of cold prevention] as a mere joke." Although he did not describe conditions in his own plant, his comments do suggest that he recognized a relationship between working conditions and health.[24] Other participants in the chamber's campaign looked even closer to the workplace for causes. One department store manager blamed drafts, while others bluntly stated that employers would do better by their employees if they paid attention to ventilation, humidity, and temperature in the plant.[25]

In an age of increased public scrutiny from state factory inspectors as well as increased attention to workers' compensation liability, businesses began to implement specific actions aimed at lowering their costs in industrial accidents. They also adopted a number of measures less evidently related to industrial accidents and illness. Contemporaries called such measures "industrial welfare" or "industrial betterment," and many historians have characterized these policies as a means to reduce labor unrest. From the perspective of occupational health, these measures also illustrate the ways in which employers and workers alike recognized that home and workplace overlapped. Formerly private family responsibilities and activities could now be handled at the factory. The installation of dining rooms and recreation areas suggests some understanding of the relationship between nutrition, fitness, and health, but businesses also established savings-and-loan facilities for employees, installed libraries and music rooms, and offered sewing clubs and English classes, activities less directly related to health.[26]

In Pittsburgh, H.J. Heinz went to great lengths to promote its canning factory as both machine and home. "Neither noise nor friction," said one manager, interfered with the company's smooth operations, and no worker's job overlapped another's. According to the same manager, however, "There is something here more than energy—there is an abundant good humor, a keen and earnest interest in, and love for, the work." He went on to describe Heinz's family-like atmosphere and the common interests of workers and managers. Heinz carried the family motif beyond descriptions of the workplace, offering classes "in all the accomplishments of the housewife."[27]

Many businesses began to provide on-site industrial nurses and physicians, who functioned almost as social workers. Brighton Mills in Passaic, New Jersey, in 1913 employed a nurse to visit workers at home for personal or family illness. Barcale Manufacturing in Buffalo, New York, went further, sending its female "welfare worker" directly into employees' homes, where she urged workers to "overcome habitual tardiness," adopt good hygiene habits, and improve their living conditions. Marshall Field, which offered a variety of on-the-job services, professed great interest in learning about the "health conditions and the influence for good or bad that are entering into [workers'] lives while absent from business."[28]

Heinz's managers stressed the plant's cleanliness while making distinctly unfavorable comparisons to workers' personal habits and living conditions. Heinz required uniforms, for instance, but did not allow workers to change into them at home. Instead, they changed in company locker rooms. By taking aim at bad living conditions, employers may not have hoped to escape all blame for the ill health of workers, but they could at least propose to share it. "By far the greater part of sickness," claimed Metropolitan Life's assistant medical director, Wade Wright, "is not produced definitely by industrial conditions, except in a very general way, because industrial workers live in an industrial age, and in an industrial era." "Reasonably good working conditions" was a loose term, he said. No amount of effort could turn "glue factories, blast furnace plants [and] coal mines . . . into little heavens."[29]

A few business owners tried to avoid all responsibility for their workers' health. Welfarism, wrote Charles H. Hulburd of Elgin Watch (Illinois), took away the workers' freedom of choice. The most intelligent employees, he said, would rather collect higher wages, "which would permit them, as free American citizens, to spend the money individually as they thought for their own best good." Royal Worcester Corset (Massachusetts) agreed. It had no fixed programs, according to E. Seward, but gave workers the tools with which to create their own welfare.[30]

While rejecting specific welfare programs as charity, E. L. Nazro of Plymouth Cordage (Massachusetts) nevertheless believed in an environmentalist trickle-down theory. He argued that a clean and tidy factory exterior, with well-kept lawns and roads, would do more for workers than welfare. (It would presumably create clean and tidy-looking workers who cleaned up their own houses and streets.) Plymouth Cordage offered prizes for the best-kept houses and yards.[31]

Were business owners influenced by gender in the introduction of welfare measures? Quite possibly, especially if we consider the actions of department stores like John Wanamaker, Filene's, and Marshall Field's, all of which installed dining rooms and rest rooms but also offered medical services and classes on vocational and cultural topics for their largely female workforce. Attention to women employees' needs had always been more acceptable than attention to men's, a point not missed by many proponents of protective labor legislation.[32]

Did businesses operate within the same worldview as reformers? Yes, insofar as both recognized the significance of the overlap between home and workplace. But their goals differed.[33] Social reformers could identify with business measures that acknowledged the interaction between home and workplace, but a close examination of the environmental measures taken by business suggests different motives. In the interests of efficiency and profitability, many businesses felt they needed to shape or control their workers' private lives. In the ever brighter spotlight trained on urban, industrial working conditions, industrial welfare strategies also offered employers a way to deflect some of their responsibility for workers' health by pointing out, through the activities of people like Barcale's welfare worker, the workers' bad living conditions and unhealthful personal habits. This practice grew more popular over time and became tied to workers' compensation legislation.[34] Reformers did not stray from their environmental position, but they did begin to consider strategies that resembled business's increasingly specialized production methods. Such strategies had a significant impact on occupational health.

During the Progressive Era, the U.S. middle class became increasingly interested in specialization. Robert Wiebe attributes structural changes in the United States at the turn of the twentieth century to an assertive middle class seeking to gain a toehold in the American power structure by professional occupation or business acumen. By stressing legitimacy based on merit and knowledge, this new class tried to dislodge more traditional credentials of power—ethnic association, family ties, wealth. According to Wiebe, the middle classes actively entered and sought to elevate such fields as medicine, law, journalism, teaching, and government into professions ruled by self-determined standards, specialization, and restriction. In government, for instance, the wide use of civil service examinations presumably determined "merit."[35]

On the one hand, the ideology of knowledge and expertise promoted efficiency and order in a confusing and complex world. Informed by rational, scientific approaches that both disaggregated problems and assumed that solving the pieces solved the whole, middle-class professionals argued that society needed specialized, reductionist knowledge to prosper. They agreed to assume the responsibility for supplying such expertise if society would, in turn, defer to their judgment.[36]

On the other hand, overcrowded cities, increasingly populated by large numbers of immigrants, touched a humanitarian chord among many in the middle class. The slums exacerbated a number of social problems—health, housing, working conditions—that often had common causes and solutions. Humanitarian Progressivism's central theme was the child—the "carrier of tomorrow's hope"—whose life was expected to be better than his or her parents'. In order to safeguard that future, urbanites who had come to depend on government for basic services demanded that it provide opportunities and promote progress. With efficiently managed policies, Progressive reformers began to apply the specialized language and principles of the period to their humanitarian goals of improving working women's lives.[37]

Specialization also occurred in the biological sciences. Changes in the medical profession were precipitated by and reflected significant discoveries. With the advent of germ theory and the technology that enabled physicians and scientists to view what had been previously invisible, more became known about the human body at the cellular level. As a result, medical treatment became more specialized, as did the medical profession. During the first years of the twentieth century, a number of medical specialties developed, including industrial medicine.[38]

As a medical philosophy, germ theory created new problems even as it solved old ones, as can be seen in the treatment of occupational diseases. Despite the increased adoption of specific measures and more advocacy for changes in the workplace, social workers and medical professionals who treated workers on a daily basis sometimes needed practical solutions to occupation-related health problems. Those answers did not always fall within the parameters of scientific medicine and its emphasis on treating discrete symptoms.

Historians of public health have noted a similar accommodation. Judith Walzer Leavitt and John Duffy have argued that even when germs had displaced filth as the explanatory cause of disease, public health reformers continued to emphasize measures to clean up poor neighborhoods. During the first years of this century, many public health activists remained wedded to changing the environment, although medical knowledge indicated that the key to solving disease lay in ridding individuals of germs. Medical and social work staffers who worked to reduce the health risks associated with working conditions also understood that the workplace environment made people sick.[39]

Boston's Massachusetts General Hospital, like other urban hospitals, had long been funded by accident-plagued corporations in exchange for treating their workers for industrial injuries. Attention to industrial diseases increased in 1907, after the passage of legislation requiring the Board of Health to establish and maintain a list of diseases dangerous to public health.[40]

Massachusetts General established its Industrial Clinic in 1912, after several years of having physicians in various departments at the hospital (including skin, nerve, dental, and orthopedic) treat patients for a number of what turned out to be work-related diseases and accidents. Prior to the creation of the clinic, the outpatient director, Dr. Richard C. Cabot, had introduced a new medical professional, the medical social worker, who ensured patient follow-through on treatments and recommendations made by medical staff. It made little sense to Cabot to treat diseases outside the context of patients' lives. "Our treatment," he said, "must be based on the recognition of two closely inter-related factors: the medical diagnosis . . . [and] the social diagnosis. . . . In making up our plan for each patient we must consider him just as he is, i.e., set in a background made up of his environment (domestic, industrial, racial) and his available resources." His support for a medical social service department underscored his belief that busy clinic physicians too often ignored the social background of patients' lives.[41]

What Cabot described, and criticized, was the growing tendency of physicians to focus on specific symptoms—often at the expense of other, nonmedical factors. Massachusetts General's head social worker, Ida Cannon, recalled seeing a young woman referred from the Female Medical Clinic because she could not afford to pay for the pills that the clinic physician prescribed for her anemia. Cannon, noticing the young woman's small size for her twenty years, began talking with her and discovered that the woman worked in a raincoat factory as a seam sealer. Fumes from the naphtha cement she used filled the air of the building where she worked and took away her appetite. "It was obvious," said Cannon, "that this patient needed more than Blaud's pills" (the iron pills prescribed for the anemia). Despite the development of casework methods in the twentieth-century social work profession, Cannon's own work remained environmentally focused. She also knew that the overlap between working women's work and domestic responsibilities created health hazards.[42]

Although medical social workers had little if any authority to change conditions in the workplace, they often used individual, practical strategies to alter a patient's working environment. After the hospital dermatologist told one young woman that her skin condition (erythema nodosum) would not improve as long as she continued to work as a waitress, the social work staff secured new employment for her at the hospital. Her skin troubles disappeared. Another young woman, overworked as a domestic for a large Boston family, received similar treatment. After arranging for a month's rest at a Boston convalescent home, the social service department found the woman a new—and presumably less fatiguing—position with the family of one of Massachusetts General Hospital's outpatient physicians.[43]

Ida Cannon's interest in the raincoat sealer and her subsequent conversations with the referring physician, Roger Lee, prompted the two of them to undertake an eight-month study of eighty "working girls" who had applied for medical relief at Massachusetts General Hospital in 1910–11. In an age of factory inspections, housing inspections, and increased studies of occupational diseases, wrote Lee, it was important to investigate the reasons behind the illnesses of these working women. Expressing the same maternalist sentiments found among advocates of protective labor legislation, Lee argued that he was concerned about the women's "present health and efficiency" only to the extent that it influenced their future health and efficiency as mothers.[44]

Partly in response to Cannon's and Lee's work, Cabot and a colleague, David Edsall, formally established the hospital's Industrial Clinic, whose mission was to consolidate, organize, and quantify the treatment of occupational diseases in the city. That the environmentalist aspects of medicine initially drove this interest is indicated by the clinic's earliest methods of attracting patients: Susan Holton, a trained nurse, positioned herself at the front door of the Outpatient Department, interviewed every patient and immediately referred likely looking cases—that is, those who worked in a growing but increasingly specific list of industries—to the Industrial Clinic. She also referred those who looked sick. The clinic's starting point was the workers' environment. As diagnosis became better targeted, this would change.[45]

The early attention paid by Massachusetts General to industrial origins of disease, particularly to the interaction between environment and health, was important because it provided a medical context for protective labor legislation. At the same time, Massachusetts General's experiences showed how specialization and environmentalism could coexist even though the medical profession emphasized specialization. The fact is, concern over women's working conditions derived from an environmentalist perspective of health and disease. Factory investigators witnessed the connection between bad working conditions and bad health; understood the blurred distinctions between home and workplace, especially for women; and believed that mothers provided the means by which the health of the next generation was established. Specific legislative actions to enact gender-based protective labor legislation most commonly centered on the need for shorter hours for working women and on their exclusion from many night jobs. Some reformers went further, arguing that mothers should be prohibited from working altogether: working mothers not only bore unhealthy children, ran the argument, they also neglected them, causing "illiteracy, delinquency, dependence."[46]

But scientific medicine continued to gain favor, and many proponents of protective labor legislation believed they needed to move beyond a strictly environmentalist position. The combination of strategies medical social workers used is similar to reformers' actions. A handful of states had enacted restrictions on women's hours of wage work by the turn of the century. State courts had upheld their legality and reaffirmed traditional notions about the primacy of women's maternal duties. A Pennsylvania Superior Court judge supported his state's sixty-hour week, twelve-hour day law for women with the comment that the "mothers of our race" should be prevented from being "tempted to endanger their life and health by exhaustive employment." But an Oregon laundry owner, Curt Muller, challenged his state's legislation limiting women's hours of work, and his case reached the U.S. Supreme Court in 1908.[47]

At that point Louis Brandeis and Josephine Goldmark, of the National Consumers' League, longtime supporters of protective labor legislation, went into high gear. They recruited ten volunteer researchers who devoted two full weeks to data-collecting from a variety of sources. Brandeis and Goldmark presented to the Court national and international examples of the deleterious effects of long hours on health, safety, morals, and general welfare. Although they relied on statistics and expert opinions from physicians, public health officials, and government watchdogs, their arguments also underscored a willingness to apply the term "hazardous" to a number of industrial conditions, combining an environmental understanding of health with the more specialized methods of modern science. They argued that women were physically different from men and were therefore more seriously fatigued by the strain of modern industry's long hours. Perhaps most persuasively, they pointed to the increased risks women faced in childbirth. The Supreme Court agreed, concluding in *Muller v. Oregon* that a "woman's physical structure and the performance of maternal functions place her at a disadvantage in the struggle for subsistence. . . . This is especially true when the burdens of motherhood are upon her." More significant, the Court affirmed that women's health was an appropriate concern for the state because it was in the public interest to "preserve the strength and vigor of the race."[48]

Protective legislation was blatantly selective, as its feminist opponents would later point out. In Pennsylvania, legislators felt free to ignore medical evidence when it inconvenienced them. After all, they might not get clean shirts if they did not allow laundries to work their women employees overtime during holiday weeks. Alice Hamilton dryly noted, in a speech at the 1917 Pennsylvania Industrial Welfare and Efficiency Conference, that the work done by tens of thousands of women who scrubbed floors and clothes belied the assumption that women were inherently weaker than men. Some working women fought protective labor laws from the very start. In 1914, for example, women printers in New York City rejected efforts by the Women's Trade Union League to shorten their hours and to prohibit them from working nights, both of which would eliminate them from many of the more highly skilled and better-paying jobs.[49]

Nevertheless, a broad coalition of activists and reformers across the country used *Muller* to push for hours restrictions, prohibition of night work, and other protective policies based on gender. By 1916 forty-two states and Puerto Rico had some form of protective labor legislation, citing both medical and social necessity. Jurisdictions with restrictions already in place continued to adjust women's maximum weekly hours downward, as Pennsylvania did in 1913, from sixty to fifty-four hours. At the same time the state established minimal sanitary requirements.[50]

The combined weight of testimony from a number of medical experts and the use of statistics and methodical research gathering constituted a conscious effort to bring the weight of modern science to bear on an important social issue, an increasingly popular Progressive strategy. In *Muller* very specific methods were used to support environmentalist goals—goals that placed responsibility for health on the workplace rather than the worker.[51] Josephine Goldmark went on to incorporate the national and international testimony that she had gathered for *Muller* into a massive study of fatigue. Published in 1912, *Fatigue and Efficiency: A Study in Industry* attempted to persuade businesses of the need for protective labor legislation by linking fatigue to industrial inefficiency. Goldmark's strategy derived from her years of involvement with the National Consumers' League, an organization devoted to improving working women's lives through economic and public pressure on employers. Her ties to the league, which lasted until her death in 1950, also indicate the league's willingness to adopt modern scientific methods to advance broader social goals.[52]

Fatigue, of course, was not a new diagnosis, nor did it exclusively derive from industrial causes—although it *was* almost exclusively applied to females. Nineteenth-century health reformers created a number of spas and rest cures as a middle-class respite from the hurried, frenetic, industrializing world. Tonics and therapies "cured" fatigue and neurasthenia. Many of these treatments represented a reaction against the often harsh "heroic" methods of formally trained physicians, promising more naturalistic, gentler therapies.[53]

Fatigue, with its visible symptoms that manifested themselves in a variety of ways and in a number of organs and muscles, easily fit into an environmentalist view of medicine, and it often seemed related to the external environment. Fatigue began to be linked to working-class health in the latter half of the nineteenth century, when the introduction of new and larger machinery spurred the drive for increased production that in turn often translated into longer working hours.

In the first years of Massachusetts General's Social Service Department, physicians often diagnosed "general debility," for which they recommended rest or sometimes iron pills. *Fatigue and Efficiency* contained hundreds of excerpts from national and international labor boards, organizations, and medical professionals attesting to the deleterious effects of long hours on women's general health, morality, mortality, family life, recreation, and reproduction. Goldmark also analyzed the new strains of industry: speed and complexity, monotony, noise, fatigue and industrial accidents, rhythm, piecework, and overtime, with special attention to new occupations for women. Goldmark pointed out that young women needed time to develop intellectual interests and to pursue recreational activities; she also warned of reproductive dangers as a result of overwork. The three visible effects of overstrain on women, according to Goldmark, were increased infant mortality, a decreased birthrate, and an "impaired second generation." Goldmark stressed the importance of environmental influences. She acknowledged that "many factors besides overwork contribute[d] to the greater mortality of infants among the working class, such as improper feeding and overcrowding," but the relationship between women's industrial work and a high death rate among infants was, in her opinion, well established.[54]

Goldmark presented U.S. and European laboratory studies on animals to illustrate the effects of repetitive motion, long periods of uninterrupted activity, and judicious use of rest periods. Adopting the methods of modern science and medicine, she studied the relationship between certain movements and their physiological consequences on specific parts of the body. Her work included graphs that depicted diminishing muscle capacity over time, with special attention to effects on productivity.[55]

Goldmark used science to emphasize the physiological aspects of fatigue and believed that changing working conditions and hours would eliminate the problem. Again reformers and business shared strategies, for business leaders also used science. They considered fatigue a psychological condition not caused by the workplace. In the years just before and during World War I, many subscribed to Frederick Winslow Taylor's vision of the workplace, where each task would be so scientifically suited to workers in terms of speed and the specific movements that, instead of experiencing fatigue, workers would "thrive while working at this rate during a long term of years and grow happier and more prosperous, instead of being overworked." Under this scenario, fatigue did not exist, so a tired-looking worker was presumably just being lazy. According to Alan Derickson, many Progressives adopted Taylorism as a legitimate method of increasing efficiency. Goldmark remained wary. While acknowledging that changes made by efficiency engineers could improve speed without creating worker fatigue, she also noted that significant fatigue was caused simply by overlong hours and employer-induced speedups.[56]

The efforts by business to shift the responsibility for maintaining the health of workers from employer to worker was one indicator of the future direction of occupational health. Labor leaders inadvertently handed employers another way to escape responsibility when they helped outlaw the suck shuttle in Massachusetts textile factories. In the humid, unventilated weaving rooms of New England cotton manufacturing establishments, tuberculosis found a hospitable environment, and the disease was endemic to the mills. Yet efforts by public health officials, employers, and labor in the early 1900s to reduce tuberculosis focused not on improving the entire work environment but on a single item—the method of threading shuttles. Women weavers drew the thread through the eye of the shuttle "by placing the shuttle to the mouth and drawing the breath," according to an 1884 description.[57] By using new medical evidence on the tubercle bacillus, which indicated that tuberculosis was spread through close personal contact, the unions successfully demanded in 1911 that the legislature ban the use of the suck shuttle. Ironically, however, the ban also allowed employers, with union and state support, to avoid changing conditions in the mills. Instead they were able to establish policy based on the notion that disease was caused by individuals, not the environment.[58]

Medical ideas do not exist in a vacuum. Older notions of medicine carried political, economic, social, and moral implications that continued to inform the workplace, particularly the workplace of women, in the early years of the twentieth century, even after germ theory had begun to displace environmental theories of disease. The visible effects of a dirty environment on maternal and family health, the blurred lines between home and factory, the virtually unquestioned primacy of a woman's domestic responsibilities—all of these helped maintain a vision that resisted modern reductionist thinking. Moreover, medicine and science interacted with and responded to prevailing ideas about gender, business, and civic practices. These ideas were supported politically by urban middle-class women's assertion of a public life, albeit within the context of more private roles. The notion of "municipal housekeeping" metaphorically extended the boundaries of home into the public arena. Business owners also tried to acknowledge the relationship between home and work by introducing traditionally private activities into the workplace.[59]

Fears about the health of women workers grew out of and reflected an environmentalist view of the world, but the intellectual shift toward specificity did not result in the demise of environmentalism. In fact, the coexistence of old and new with respect to the occupational health of women helped legitimate reformers' agenda.

Not unlike public health activists who used modern notions about germ theory to promote sanitary reforms (even as they had previously called for cleaner cities based on filth theories of medicine), reformers initially believed that this coexistence promised and provided new methods of supporting the original goals of cleaning up the workplace and achieving better health for working women.[60] Specialized research on respiratory diseases, for instance, provided "proof" of the need for better ventilation. The adoption of modern science later reduced the physical dimensions of the workplace environment to individual boundaries, but in the early years of the twentieth century, reformers used modern research to support broad-based environmental reform. An equally broad characterization of women's maternal roles modified medicine's impact on occupational health for men and women. For working women, protective legislation supported women's broadly defined social roles as mothers. Legislation focused on the big picture, and reformers did not study or consider the actual variations in women's lives and the individual choices they made to provide material and maternal care for their families.

2

Industrial Poisons:
The Two-Percent Solution

When Alice Hamilton spoke before Pennsylvania's Industrial Welfare and Efficiency Conference in 1917, she praised the increased entrance of women into nontraditional jobs in industry but expressed a popular reservation about such moves: "It will be no boon to women if it demands that they are to enter trades which are not fitted for them and do work which will injure their health." To Hamilton the protection of women was important, although she qualified her position: "I am myself in favor of employing women in all such work so long as the danger is not one to which her sex is peculiarly liable; so long as the danger is one which a man faces equally, I think there is no reason why a woman should not face it also."[1]

Hamilton's particular expertise was industrial poisons; she feared that some industrial materials such as lead interfered with or inhibited women's ability to bear children. Despite mounting evidence from Hamilton and other physicians that hazards like lead were "race poisons"—substances with serious reproductive implications for motherhood and the next generation—state labor agencies and legislatures largely expressed their pro-natalism only through efforts to reduce women's hours in the workplace.

Support for limiting the hours of women was based on a broad understanding of what constituted a hazardous environment. A longer workday for women risked social harm because it increased fatigue at home, corrupted the morals of children left without supervision, and threatened women's ability to be good mothers. Night work contributed to low morals in women. The risks associated with industrial poisons, however, were limited to physical harm: exposure to lead was bad because it produced physiological changes that interfered with or damaged women's ability to bear healthy children. Women's capacity for motherhood provided the rationale for both kinds of protection; women's traditional responsibility for reproducing the race justified protection.

Hamilton's distinction between harm caused by excessive hours and harm based on reproductive dangers reflects a small, but in retrospect significant, inclination toward biology, not social norms, in determining workplace boundaries. While the use of reproductive knowledge to define women's health antedated the twentieth century, the combination of modern medicine, increasingly specific methods of defining workplace health and safety, and what Nancy Cott has called "modern feminism" prompted a shift toward a more narrow construction of gender roles that would theoretically widen women's work opportunities.

By the second half of the nineteenth century, physicians had increased their attention to female reproduction, seeking to connect women more tightly to the biological bonds of maternity. Carroll Smith-Rosenberg and others have attributed these concerns to middle-class white women's improving economic and educational opportunities, marked in part by a declining birthrate. Women's attempts to control their own fertility, writes Smith-Rosenberg, resulted in, among other things, restrictions on the dissemination of information on contraception and in laws against abortion. The American Medical Association in particular criticized middle-class women's "unnatural" autonomy and accused these women of "self-indulgence": "She yields to the pleasures—but shrinks from the pains and responsibilities of maternity." James Reed, in his history of birth control in the United States, attributed these restrictions to male fear of middle-class women's dissatisfaction with domesticity. According to Reed, the source of this fear lay in the increasingly self-conscious medical profession's belief in its own responsibility to maintain traditional social order. Linda Gordon likewise noted the relationship between physicians' professional goals and their belief in "lowering birth rates *selectively* [emphasis in original]," that is, among the immigrant and working classes. This agenda had replaced earlier activism by nineteenth-century feminists on behalf of "voluntary motherhood."[2]

Scientists, psychologists, and social observers, also concerned about declining birth and marriage rates, feared that higher education for women resulted in what the physician Edward Clarke called "undeveloped ovaries." With an understanding of health based on the moderation of energy expenditure, the psychologist G. Stanley Hall supported Clarke's hypothesis with statistics of his own on graduates of women's colleges like Vassar, Smith, and Wellesley. All the figures confirmed Herbert Spencer's argument that "absolute or relative infertility is generally produced in women by any mental labor carried to excess." College-educated women married less frequently than women with less education. Cynthia Russett appropriately placed these attempts to control women's lives through their reproductive abilities as a last gasp, an "intellectual monument, etched in fear, of the painful transition to the modern world view."[3] Their attitudes also provided a social and scientific context for shifts in the definition of motherhood toward its biological characteristics.

During this period, childbirth, which had long been presided over by midwives and birthing women, was coopted by the medical profession, taking reproductive control out of the hands of women. By the turn of the twentieth century, the growth of medical knowledge threatened to separate women from their birthing experiences.[4] The process of transforming birth into a medical rather than a female-centered social event had turned childbirth into nothing more than a biological activity.

Similarly, treatments for infertility and a variety of conditions associated with female reproduction became less the province of midwives and more of physicians in the new specialty of gynecology. During this same period, according to Margaret Marsh and Wanda Ronner, gynecologists physically separated women from their reproductive functions altogether by surgically removing the ovaries, citing any number of symptoms to justify the procedure. The development of surgical techniques and mechanical devices promised to keep gynecologists in control of reproductive functions indefinitely.[5]

Despite scientific interest in women's reproductive abilities during this period, few used the new knowledge to challenge prevailing notions about motherhood. In fact, gynecologists used science to reinforce the belief that all diseases of women "originated in their reproductive organs." Even female social reformers who led nontraditional lives stressed the primacy of women's domestic responsibilities. Most social reformers who sought to control working-class women did so through their belief in traditional gender norms, characterized by broad social and maternal roles and by women's devotion to family and community. Not surprisingly, these beliefs surfaced in public health efforts directed at helping the working class rear healthy children. In cities across the United States, both volunteers and paid professionals, largely female, took part in a variety of "baby-saving" projects, from pure milk campaigns to "little mothers' classes" to providing skilled nursing care for infants. Aimed at immigrant working-class mothers, these programs sought not only to reduce infant mortality rates but also to Americanize these women with lessons in proper maternal roles. Reformers believed that being a mother often meant performing a wide variety of tasks—child-rearing, housework, and community relations—many of which went well beyond the comparatively narrow task of bearing a child.[6]

Efforts by social workers to get single mothers to keep their children, for instance, exemplify not only moral prescriptions about women's need to live with the wages of their sin but also attitudes about the redemptive quality of motherhood. A single mother, according to the social worker Ida Cannon, would "get out of motherhood all the wisdom and joy that every mother should get out of it" through the rearing of her children. These mothers' devotion to such children, of course, with the help of social workers and family members, would ensure adequate living conditions to provide for the children's health needs. For social workers motherhood included any number of social and cultural tasks, and in many ways, biology actually seemed *less* important than these.[7]

Against the backdrop of this broad construction of early twentieth-century maternalism, the introduction of chemical substances into the workplace threatened to expose men and women workers to a variety of new dangers that would force workers and labor officials to rely increasingly on medical expertise. The struggle over how best to fix the workplace occurred within relatively narrow boundaries, initially in the context of a small but developing interest in the biological components of motherhood, as exemplified by attitudes toward chemicals like lead and benzene. The interest in working-class women's biological capacity to reproduce belies much of the contemporary and secondary literature on race suicide, which has tended to focus on criticism of middle-class women's unwillingness to reproduce and working-class women's willingness to reproduce too frequently. Reformers with an interest in working women's biological health seem to have ignored warnings about working-class fecundity.[8]

Material conditions in the second half of the nineteenth century had prompted serious attention to the workplace.[9] Efforts to protect workers from industrial injury and illness received new impetus in the late nineteenth century as courts began to strike down traditional employer defenses against workers' charges of negligence. David Rosner and Gerald Markowitz have argued that a broad coalition of writers, physicians, social workers, and consumer activists emphasized the need to change the workplace environment and control the chemicals and poisons that had become a regular part of the twentieth-century workplace.[10]

One significant problem revolved around the containment of hazardous materials to the specific area of the factory using them. For instance, lead was and is still an important material in the making of batteries. In contrast to claims that hazardous materials could be spatially confined, a 1912 investigation of a Niagara Falls plant found lead everywhere. "In nearly every branch of production," charged George Price, "there was a large amount of lead dust and fumes, the floors were saturated with lead dust, and tests of the air in the various parts of the plant clearly showed amounts of lead . . . to cause serious injury."[11]

Hamilton agreed with Price's dismal description of U.S. factories. She had long praised European achievements in the protection of workers, after being forced to agree with the assessment given at an international gathering of occupational health professionals in 1911 that "there is no industrial hygiene in the United States. Ça n'existe pas." Europe had established strict rules on dangerous trades, including the white-lead trade, as early as 1898, and Hamilton considered England to have the "highest standard in factory inspection and legal protection of the workers." David Edsall likewise praised France's successful regulation of the white-lead trade, which resulted in fewer cases of lead poisoning in Paris in two years than he saw at Episcopal Hospital in Philadelphia in

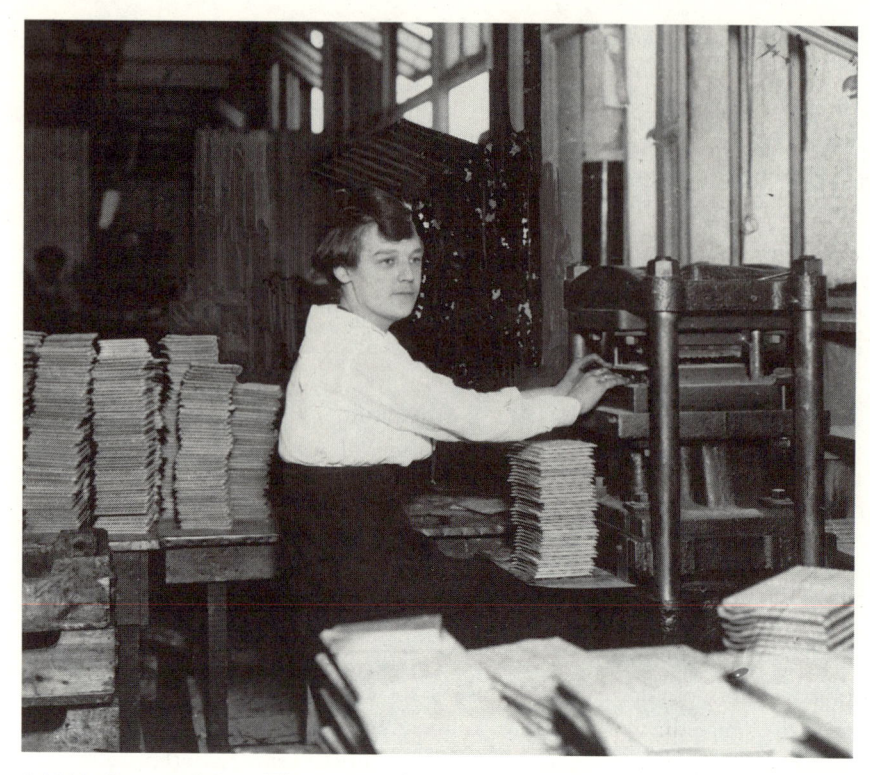

A 1919 photograph from Thomas A. Edison and Co. of a woman worker stamping out lead plates for Edison Storage Batteries, despite legislation in New Jersey that restricted women's exposure to lead.

one. U.S. health reformers moved more slowly than their European counterparts, but in the early twentieth century, a multiclass and multi-interest movement successfully raised the awareness of industrialization's deleterious effects on workers, including their exposure to lead.[12]

Lead had long been recognized as a hazard to industrial workers. Charles Dickens in 1869 vividly described lead poisoning's characteristic "wrist drop" paralysis, chronic weakness, and pallid complexion in a female character in *The Uncommercial Traveler—All the Year Round:* "Better [for her] to be ulcerated and paralyzed for eighteen pence a day . . . than see the children starve."[13]

Of the two major kinds of lead poisoning—acute and chronic—the chronic variety was far more common in the United States at the turn of the century. Hamilton's analysis of lead poisoning in the 1910s indicates a series of physiological changes nearly identical to those detailed in 1973 handbooks on occupational health hazards. Chronic lead poisoning lowers resistance to disease by rupturing red blood cells. This also leads to the degeneration of organs, especially the kidneys. Lead can also affect the nervous system by hardening the arteries in the brain. Many physicians, including Hamilton, initially believed that fewer hours of exposure would give the worker's body sufficient time to recover from the effects of lead, but further research indicated that lead remains in the body for some time after exposure.[14]

Many U.S. industries—lead mining, smelting and refining, printing, grinding paint, painting, manufacturing storage batteries, and glazing pottery—exposed workers to lead. Reports by U.S. health officials on lead poisoning began to appear in the first decade of this century, although the published medical research on lead, except for Hamilton's, remained heavily foreign for a number of years. Only a few British physicians—Sir Thomas Oliver, for example—seem to have been read in the United States.[15]

Organic poisons like coal tar benzene did not appear on the U.S. industrial scene until World War I, when the small supply of benzene from Germany was cut off. Because benzene's high volatility made it a crucial element in the manufacture of explosives, its demand greatly increased during the war. After the war, manufacturers searched for new markets, which they found in rubber and leather industries, for benzene was an excellent solvent. Manufacturers of sanitary cans, such as those used in food processing, liked the cementing properties of benzene. It was also used somewhat later for cementing wood heels to leather shoes. Benzene is a volatile solvent that, if inhaled or ingested, causes bone marrow failure: it reduces the blood's clotting ability and iron levels, producing excessive bleeding and anemia. It also causes liver damage.[16]

One of the more notable instances of early industrial poisoning in this country occurred in the match industry at the turn of the century. Physicians became aware that white phosphorus caused necrosis of the jaw, commonly known as "phossy jaw." Angela Nugent has described how the furor over phossy jaw resulted in the elimination of white phosphorus from the industry. For most industrial hazards, however, elimination or substitution was not an option, although employers did occasionally develop substitutes.[17]

Many labor reformers believed it was industry's responsibility to eliminate hazardous chemicals from the workplace. Industrialists, however, preferred control, which could be defined by measurement and statute, to elimination. In their efforts to predict business costs, employers supported the passage of workers' compensation laws, which obligated employers to pay insurance premiums based on industry-wide accident rates. They relied on experts to pinpoint specific problem areas inside the plant and to suggest specific solutions. Blowers and exhaust hoods for ventilation, as well as devices to measure precise concentrations of poisons, usually noted in parts per million, became common pieces of equipment in factories. In the interests of limiting liability, companies also increasingly tried to shift responsibility to individual workers for maintaining personal cleanliness.[18]

Many physicians agreed with industry's efforts. One complained that workers who did not wash their hands before eating caused preventable occupational diseases. Even worse, he declared, they set a bad example for their children. In his opinion, employers should coerce change. In a 1911 study of working women, Roger Lee argued that many workers could improve their lot with "knowledge of the hygiene of body [and] mind."[19]

The medical profession found other reasons to support this limited approach to occupational health. Paul Starr attributes the rise of industrial medicine during this period to developments in the practice of medicine and in industrial relations. Specifically, medical journals began to emphasize the importance of preventive health care, and many industrialists relied heavily on the scientific management theories of Frederick Taylor.[20] Industrial medicine quickly attracted doctors in city hospitals who were treating increasing numbers of occupational accidents. The research possibilities suggested by the growing evidence of more-difficult-to-diagnose occupational diseases also prompted hospitals to establish industrial disease clinics. After Massachusetts General established its Industrial Disease Clinic in 1912, staff members soon found themselves developing and distributing "Advice to Persons Working with Lead" and "Precautions for Printers." Professor Alfred Stengel established a clinic at the hospital of the University of Pennsylvania's medical school in 1916. The passage of occupational disease reporting laws such as those in New Jersey and Pennsylvania in 1912 and 1913, respectively, forced physicians to educate themselves about the symptoms of the diseases whose incidence they were required to report. The need for continuing professional education resulted in annual conferences about occupational health and disease, the first of which was held in 1914.[21]

Despite the attraction of specialization, however, government officials in the early years of factory inspections resisted narrowly defining their responsibilities. The initial factory inspection laws had targeted women and children, so industrial states necessarily defined hazards rather broadly. Relying on traditional notions about women's domestic responsibilities, inspectors believed they had an obligation to identify a broad array of dangerous workplace conditions, all of which had a deleterious effect on home and family. Moreover, inspectors interpreted their responsibilities to reach beyond merely ensuring women's and children's health and safety. Concerned about conditions for all workers, they often used the factory inspection law as a means of learning about factory conditions in general.[22]

State officials relied on medical experts but also acknowledged their own expertise as they became more involved in developing mechanical devices to improve workplace conditions, issued health and safety regulations for many occupations, and even established museums of safety. Within two years of its creation, the Pennsylvania Department of Labor and Industry Industrial Board was regularly publishing "Timely Hints" for workers in certain industries. In addition it had issued seventeen mandatory codes, most of them dealing with safety. New Jersey inspectors systematically investigated different industries. They exhibited a degree of self-consciousness, no doubt strengthened by the new civil service status of their jobs and informed by the department's desire to upgrade standards in order to attract a "high grade of young men" to the positions, although they still relied on the volunteer efforts of "eight public-spirited ladies" as late as 1912.[23]

Just as in their battles after *Muller v. Oregon*, reformers faced narrower interpretations of occupational disease. Many who sought to improve workplace health needed new methods. Their environmentalist approach had its limits. First, they often failed to consider medical evidence that not all workers exposed to the same chemical experienced symptoms, suggesting differences in individual susceptibility. Also, their insistence on considering the overlap between home and work made it hard to pin illness exclusively on the workplace. Finally, and most important to those who favored state intervention and the regulation of industrial hazards, the environmentalist approach lacked a firm scientific basis for negotiation with industry, whose experience in and emphasis on safety measures provided a more reductionist, measurable model. In order to make an impact, environmentalist reformers needed to adopt the new, narrow vocabulary and methods.

Activists insisted that it was the state's duty to furnish employers with expert advice about changing industrial methods. As a result, while protective labor legislation in the form of shorter hours had evolved from gendered concerns about maternal health, regulations regarding industrial hazards resulted from a reliance on expert advice, which necessarily focused on the individual parts of the workplace rather than on the entire environment. For example, when the Pennsylvania legislature passed its "Woman's Law" in 1913, it did not intend to exclude women from industries that used lead in their processes; neither did the Department of Labor and Industry, which issued regulations regarding the workplace. The law specifically mandated sanitary conditions under which women could work in white-lead industries. The conditions included the provision of lunchrooms separated from the workroom, exhaust fans, and exhaust hoods above work stations. Likewise, the legislature's 1913 Lead Poisoning Law, which mandated workplace regulations and medical examinations for workers in lead industries, did not exclude women, nor did the legislature debate the issue publicly. Regulation of working conditions in hazardous industries did not evolve from concerns about maternal health even though twenty years earlier, factory inspections had been mandated on the basis of just such interests.[24]

While labor activists used the women's hours laws as an opening wedge for demanding a shorter workday for men, the same tactic did not apply in the case of occupational diseases. Pennsylvania and New Jersey did not target women in their occupational disease laws in the hope of eventually including male workers as well. The exposure of women to industrial poisons seems to have been a secondary concern, and controlling the number of hours that women spent in the workplace remained the preferred method of protecting them.[25]

World War I changed these attitudes, hastening and heightening awareness of the presence of women in dangerous trades. Wartime also heightened pronatalist thinking. Labor shortages forced industries to hire women in factories and in positions that they had not filled. State labor departments realized that shorter hours legislation alone would not sufficiently protect women from known industrial hazards. In the face of industrial pressure to lift restrictions on hours and on night work, the Pennsylvania Industrial Board tried to balance the demands of the war against traditional ideas and rules designed to protect women.[26]

Many jobs previously closed to women now exposed them to lead. This was dangerous; several centuries of experience with industrial lead exposure had left European lead industries well aware that lead poisoning adversely affected women's reproductive processes. By the late nineteenth century, a number of nations prohibited the employment of women in the lead trades. Basing her opinion on French laboratory experiments, Hamilton believed that lead damaged the "germ cells" of both men and women. But the danger to women was greater, she said, because lead circulating in the system of pregnant women affected the child "throughout its intra-uterine life." The British physician Thomas Oliver had found lead in placentas as well as in the internal organs of infants who had died. British researchers also reported 27.2 percent of housewives had had miscarriages as opposed to 74.2 percent of women who had worked with lead before marriage, and 99.0 percent of those who continued working with lead after marriage. Similarly, the number of stillbirths rose from 14.8 percent for housewives to 32.8 percent for women who worked with lead after marriage.[27]

Although physicians at that time did not know the specific ways in which lead was stored in the body other than in the blood, Oliver became alarmed that even women who quit working with lead before they became pregnant suffered a higher rate of stillbirths and miscarriages. By the early 1920s, Hamilton would begin to note lead's long-term effects on reproduction and express concerns about the lead industry's unmarried, childless women workers, in addition to its married ones.[28]

Physicians who treated or studied industrial poisons saw clear evidence that lead posed special dangers for female workers and for society. Hamilton noted the widespread belief that women were more susceptible to lead poisoning than men, but after analyzing the organization of work in the U.S. lead industries, she was skeptical. She sometimes doubted that women displayed more susceptibility than men, believing instead that poverty played a greater role than gender in predisposing to lead poisoning. Regardless of susceptibility, the most disastrous and irrefutable effect of lead exposure was on women's reproductive systems. "Lead is a race poison," she wrote. "Women who suffer from lead poisoning are more likely to be sterile or to have miscarriages and stillbirths than are women not exposed to lead." Nevertheless, she told a Pennsylvania audience in 1917, lead was the only "poison peculiarly injurious to women," and therefore the only one that women needed to be protected from in industries that manufactured white lead and storage batteries, and in the painting trades. She urged industry to concentrate on individual processes in determining women's exclusion, and offered specific suggestions in her reports and public speeches.[29]

Hamilton also tried to convince industry to look carefully at where individual employees worked within the plant. In potteries, for instance, a higher proportion of women who produced white ware got lead poisoning than did women in art potteries. More women in white ware worked directly with lead glazes, while in the art potteries, some women were engaged in non-lead processes.[30]

Armed with medical data on "race poisons" as well as its own wartime inspections, the Pennsylvania Industrial Board kept women firmly in mind in their attention to industrial processes. The board published codes and a series of rules ("Regarding Women in Industry") reflecting that orientation. Codes issued on lead corroding and oxidizing, paint grinding, and dry color industry did not exclude women from these industries but in 1917 did prohibit them from handling "any dry substance or compound containing lead in excess of 2%." New Jersey and Pennsylvania were the only states expressly prohibiting women from working with dry lead. Pennsylvania analyzed the industry further, permitting women to work on some types of production in the white-lead industry but not on others. For example, in manufacturing white lead, women could set up the lead sheets to be corroded into white lead, but they were prohibited from removing the corroded sheets after the process was completed, presumably because of the presence of large amounts of white-lead powder. Although the specificity of the codes and rules indicates that the board felt some pressure to ease restrictions on women's work during the war, it also suggests the direct influence of medical research by physicians like Hamilton and Oliver, whose recommendation on white lead in his report for the Bureau of Labor in 1911 was followed to the letter in Pennsylvania's Rule W-17.[31]

State officials in New York faced similar pressures to lift restrictions on women's work during World War I, but their experience with reproductive hazards preceded the war. The New York State Factory Investigating Commission had specifically studied the occupational health hazards affecting women workers in the context of maternity. The commission believed that women should not work in foundries, for example, because the working conditions created a danger to women as well as "a menace to posterity."[32]

Though not specifically a toxic threat to reproduction, work in foundries was increasingly understood as a physiological rather than a moral threat to motherhood. Few women worked in foundries, however, and the commission made a special effort to emphasize hazards in other, predominantly female, occupations. For example, laundry work caused pelvic problems for "body ironers," whose efforts to operate foot treadles produced a constant jerking motion. And high infant mortality, noted one investigator, might have been due as much to work during pregnancy and early return to work after birth as to specific poisons. The commissioners also paid attention to embroidery factories, for instance, where the introduction of lead powders used to mark patterns on cloth, created reproductive hazards. Workers, 80 percent of them female, in tobacco processing factories, experienced high rates of irregular menstruation, excessive menstrual bleeding, spontaneous abortions, high infant mortality, and "the bearing of weak offspring."[33]

After World War I began, the Women in Industry Service of the U.S. Department of Labor, in cooperation with the Bureau of Women in Industry of the New York State Industrial Commission, investigated industries in Niagara Falls that exposed women to "special hazards," defined as occupational dangers that affected women more seriously than men.[34]

Lead was the major hazard in Niagara Falls and was found most commonly in storage battery manufacturing companies. Investigators argued that lead posed greater hazards to women than to men not only because women were believed to be more susceptible than men to lead poisoning but also because lead caused sterility, miscarriages, and stillbirths. "For a woman," wrote Mary van Kleeck, "the poison affects not only herself but her children in the future." Echoing her friend Hamilton, however, van Kleeck, a social researcher for the Russell Sage Foundation, urged outright prohibition of women's employment only in the case of lead. Investigators made specific recommendations for cleaning up the lead battery plant—concrete floors, mechanical exhaust fans, fresh drinking water, clean company-supplied work clothes—as well as such suggestions for home hygiene as clean hands and fingernails, good health care, and a proper breakfast.[35]

Hamilton's and van Kleeck's attention to lead's reproductive hazards during the war suggests a new orientation toward state labor laws, one focusing on individual workers' characteristics and specific work processes. The two researchers used the language and methods of modern specialism in pinpointing specific tasks in industry rather than calling for blanket prohibitions against hiring women. They believed this offered women wider employment choices in industry.[36]

Like lead, benzene endangered women's reproductive abilities. Although no state acted on benzene poisoning as Pennsylvania and New Jersey did on lead, an examination of how reformers, medical professionals, business owners, and federal and state bureaucrats treated benzene as an industrial poison provides some interesting comparisons to the actions taken with respect to lead poisoning. In contrast to government action on lead poisoning, publicity and information about benzene was disseminated largely through local reform organizations, primarily the Consumers' Leagues. As in the case of lead however, reformers were careful to insist on accurate information about benzene's actual dangers, and they were reluctant to alarm unnecessarily women workers who were at risk for benzene poisoning. Studying the treatment of benzene as an industrial poison offers another opportunity to observe the evolution of this different rationale for protecting women—from concerns about working women's ability to raise children to worries about their ability to bear healthy children.

Benzene slows the production of new blood cells, reduces platelet counts, and causes internal and external hemorrhages. In many ways benzene is more dangerous than lead and more dangerous to women than to men because the consequences of exposure go beyond the reproductive. A woman's monthly menstrual cycle provided a potentially fatal site for excessive hemorrhages caused by benzene. In 1922 Hamilton and others distinguished between acute and chronic benzene poisoning, arguing that chronic poisoning was more dangerous for women than for men because of reproductive dangers, including excessive menstrual bleeding, miscarriages or, at the very least, unhealthy pregnancies.[37]

Hamilton's rationale for protecting women from benzene was identical to her stance on lead: women should not be exposed to benzene not because they were necessarily more susceptible or weaker than men, but because, "if they do suffer from the effects, they may pass the injury onto their offspring." Hamilton admitted having insufficient evidence on the specific damage done by benzene, and she was acutely aware of the dangers of making inaccurate information public. We need to be "better informed about certain puzzling features of [benzene] poisoning," she told National Consumers' League General Secretary Florence Kelley, apparently referring to disagreement over diagnosis among physicians, industry officials, academics, and state and federal industrial hygienists.[38]

Because of Hamilton's caution and her belief that remedying specific conditions would expand women's work opportunities, she supported the National Safety Council's desire to regulate the workplace and the workforce. Claudia Clark has recounted the development of an industry policy on benzene in the 1920s that advocated the exclusion of workers based on a threshold white blood cell count, as well as Hamilton's reluctant support of it. The dilemma for Hamilton was that industry's emphasis on the specific theoretically gave equal chances to male and female workers. But a single standard did not sufficiently take into account the reproductive hazards that seemed to be associated with benzene. This led Hamilton and others to continue to search for specific physiological changes caused by benzene. By 1931, for example, it was discovered that being female did not so much predispose workers to benzene poisoning as much as being young did. Moreover, a narrow definition of severe benzene poisoning, one based strictly on marrow aplasia (undeveloped stem cells, often a cause of low white blood cell counts), turns out to have disproportionately singled out women and excluded many men who exhibited hyperplastic marrow (overproduction of blood cells), which was also a "characteristic finding in many benzene cases." To Hamilton's dismay, hyperplastic anemia (anemia caused by overproduction of blood cells) apparently did not become part of the diagnosis for benzene poisoning.[39]

In the 1920s the Consumers' League of Massachusetts put great public pressure on industry to clean up its factories. In an example of grassroots rather than state action, the league undertook several industrial hazard surveys aimed at working women, including one in 1924 on women exposed to benzene in drycleaning establishments. A 1929 report published in local newspapers charged the shoe industry with poisoning many of its working women with benzene cement.[40]

The manufacture of the modern welt shoe required the use of cement rather than traditional stitching, according to shoe industry representatives. Consumers' League of Massachusetts researchers interviewed industrial officials as well as workers and former workers. Investigators also worked closely with personnel at Massachusetts General's Industrial Disease Clinic, following up suspicious cases of poisoning. Instead of being concerned with studying specific engineering methods or making environmental measurements of benzene to reduce exposure, league members urged the public to support state inspection efforts. The cleanup of the workshop, argued the league, "ultimately rests upon inspection and proper control of the workplace." The combination of local activism based on anecdotal evidence and strong support for experts gave the league the flexibility needed to retain community support from workers, the public, and industry while it pursued its broader maternalist agenda.[41]

In the meantime, Hamilton, stymied by her inability to obtain foundation money to study workplace hazards, continued to encourage state and city Consumers' Leagues to investigate industries in their areas. In 1924 the Consumers' League of Baltimore was eager to look at benzene poisoning in a local can factory. Despite Hamilton's reluctance to be caught in possible inaccuracies about benzene, she believed that grassroots activism might at least lead to factory inspection and an effective, if local, movement for a safe substitute for the chemical. In 1925 she redirected her efforts toward securing funds for the Baltimore study instead of her own, although she expressed doubts about her ability to obtain support for either project: "I have applied to the Carnegie, the Commonwealth, and the Rockefeller Foundation . . . for studies far less antagonistic to capital than this would be, and always in vain."[42]

Benzene, like lead, continued to be a part of women's industrial experiences. The U.S. Department of Labor's Women's Bureau reported on New Hampshire shoe industries in 1932, finding inadequate ventilation of benzene where it was used in cementing heels. Despite successful efforts by some can manufacturing companies to use latex as a substitute, one company feared a return to benzene after one of the largest customers of cans convinced its can supplier, the Barrett Company, that it preferred benzene-cemented cans. Bradley Dewey, of the Dewey and Almay Chemical Company, urged Hamilton to talk the Barrett Company out of the proposed switch, and he wrote to an executive at Barrett himself, defending Hamilton's "crusade" against benzene.[43]

Benzene's long-term effects had become clearer by the 1930s. A woman who pasted mica, probably in vacuum tubes, at General Electric in Schenectady, New York, stopped working with benzene in 1930 when she exhibited an "abnormal blood picture," and although the company physician wanted her to continue working in another part of the plant, he admitted that the ability to work depended on a worker's "individual constitution." The woman stopped working with benzene, received compensation for three years, yet still died at a local hospital of severe anemia characteristic of benzene poisoning. Can factory workers continued to be poisoned. In 1940 an eighteen-year-old worker from Brooklyn's Lincoln Can Factory died at King's County Hospital after bleeding vaginally for fourteen days, despite repeated transfusions.[44] Just as worrisome was the diffusion of benzene into other workplaces. Francis Hunter, a medical social worker at Massachusetts General, described a benzene-poisoned telephone operator who cleaned her switchboard each day with a small amount of paint remover.[45]

Despite the known effects of benzene on women, no state acted as Pennsylvania and New Jersey had with lead. Most action taken during this period to protect women focused on upholding and maintaining a wide array of tasks associated with motherhood, which translated into limiting women's wage-earning hours. With respect to benzene, Vilma Hunt has suggested that state inaction may have been due to the lack of evidence that it decreased fertility or harmed fetuses or infants. Workers were expendable, Hunt writes, but healthy offspring were socially valuable. She argues that the state felt reluctant to establish industrial rules if a chemical did not harm actual offspring.

The effectiveness of nongovernmental activism to garner attention and foster health and safety changes in the workplace, however, must also be considered. The Consumers' League of New Jersey's activism around radium dial painting in the 1920s illustrates the effectiveness of bringing sufficient publicity and pressure on the state and industry. In several states, women who painted watch faces and a variety of machine dials with luminescent radium for U.S. Radium Corporation suffered severe facial bone loss, painful disfigurement, and eventual death from radium poisoning. Advocacy on their behalf forced significant changes in occupational disease compensation and the industrial use of radium.[46]

In 1930 the American Public Health Association adopted lead standards for women virtually identical to those set by Pennsylvania and New Jersey, recommending the prohibition of women from jobs that required the handling of dry lead in excess of 2 percent. Lead poisoning continued to plague women, however. Indeed, whether New Jersey and Pennsylvania succeeded in substantially reducing women's risk of lead poisoning is unclear. A 1937 Department of Labor and Industry report found more than 4,500 female cases of "potential exposures to lead" in 16,000 industries. New Jersey fared little better. During World War II a Women's Bureau survey of 137 New Jersey industries still found evidence of lead exposure in female employees.[47] Industries continued to use lead, and women continued to be employed in jobs that involved handling it. In the spray enameling industry of the 1930s, employers did not consider excluding women for maternal reasons. The employment or exclusion of women was instead based on the local labor market and the size of the pieces being sprayed with leaded enamel. Hamilton worried about this new lead trade, in which gas ranges, kitchen cabinets, refrigerators, and kitchen tables were painted. Because the leaded enamel paint was in a spray gun, workers could not easily control the overspray.[48]

Industrial Poisons 43

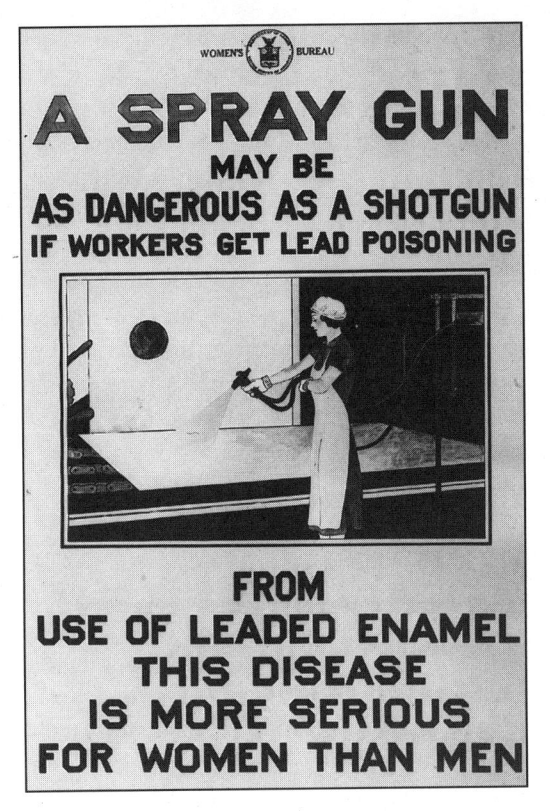

> **A SPRAY GUN MAY BE AS DANGEROUS AS A SHOTGUN IF WORKERS GET LEAD POISONING**
>
> **FROM USE OF LEADED ENAMEL THIS DISEASE IS MORE SERIOUS FOR WOMEN THAN MEN**

This Women's Bureau poster warned of the hazards of spraying lead-based enamel paint, a process introduced in the 1930s.

Subsequent investigation by the Women's Bureau revealed a significant number of single and married women with more than one symptom of lead poisoning. Because of the spraying process, Hamilton remained skeptical of effective protection other than through the substitution of leadless glazes. In the meantime, neither she nor the Women's Bureau recommended the prohibition of all women from the industry, but only those men and women who had previously been lead poisoned or who developed symptoms subsequent to employment. Hamilton suggested a variety of industrial and personal hygiene practices to improve safety. While she repeated her approval of prohibitory legislation in Pennsylvania and New Jersey, she not only understood the difference between ideal and actual practices, she also believed that paying attention to very well-designed, highly targeted engineering and health measures in this industry would sufficiently protect women workers.[49]

Early twentieth-century concerns about occupational disease developed out of two overlapping ideas about health. One relied on a broad definition of what constituted a hazardous environment; the other construed the environment more narrowly. By the 1920s government was relying more on the narrow definition, and its responsibility for ensuring a healthy workplace had diminished in proportion. State officials remained concerned about the effects of "devitalized air" on industrial workers' health, but they increasingly attacked health hazards with specific rules, regulatory processes, and specialized mechanical devices. They assigned a greater share of the responsibility to keep clean to workers, limiting the definition of "environment" to an individual worker's immediate surroundings, including his or her own body. For example, Pennsylvania's Lead Poisoning Act not only required employers to furnish workers with nail brushes, soap, and adequate washing facilities but also required employers to monitor the workers' personal habits. Industry established its own guidelines for controlling benzene, and these also regulated the worker: pre-employment examinations, for example, sought to screen out prospective employees whose white blood cell count was below 5,000, as well as those with "hemorrhagic tendencies."[50]

The increased adoption of modern medical attitudes both helped and hurt working women. On the one hand, although the notion of individual susceptibility put the burden of health on the individual rather than on industry, it also suggested a number of categories other than gender by which to determine the likelihood of illness, for example, age. Moreover, if predisposition resulted from many factors and not just from gender, women might become less industry's special victims and more simply workers. Speakers at Pennsylvania's 1925 Women in Industry conference suggested strategies for improving women's efficiency in industry, reducing fatigue, matching people with appropriate jobs, and holding workers and employers jointly responsible for industrial cleanliness. Women's perceived special health needs received little attention in state forums.[51]

On the other hand, more modern ideas did not automatically result in greater employment opportunities for women. Charles Rosenberg has argued that both old and new scientific theories can be used to validate the same social behavior—in this case the association of women with motherhood. Filth theory, for example, had justified protective labor legislation because the tendency to look at the patient in his or her entire environment resonated with those who saw women's domestic responsibilities being threatened by the time spent in the industrial environment. At the same time, scientific evidence about poisons gave new authority to those who wanted to use biology to reinforce traditional gender roles. The underlying rationale for protecting women because of their maternal capacity had survived the intellectual shift from one disease theory to another, even if in a more narrowly defined form. Although few criticized this orientation at the time, this kind of protection would become unacceptable as an employment policy for feminists and labor activists by the 1970s.[52]

Finally, workers, both male and female, used all their senses to view their surroundings, often in contrast to industry's and medicine's emphasis on the specific. In the case of vitreous enameling of stoves, some manufacturers switched to leadless glazes. Despite these improvements, however, workers remained unconvinced that the workplace was somehow healthier and attributed their sickness to dust, leaded or not. "The dust gets in your stomach and makes a hard lump; it isn't healthy," said one. Workers also recognized the ill effects of poverty. Weavers in New Jersey who worked the night shift knew that low wages, as much as hours and plant conditions, contributed to ill health. In such ways workers' understanding of the environment was becoming even more distant from industry's.[53]

3

Industrial Health in an Industrializing World

In 1926, a New York State medical inspector, Dr. Thomas O'Brien, warned workers of the tragic consequences of inattention to hygiene on the job. He described the death of an infant due, he claimed, to exposure to the father's clothes, which were contaminated with lead and aniline dye. The father frequently came home for lunch without changing his clothes, often picking his child up to greet him. Also, the mother admitted washing work clothing together with the baby's clothes. As a result, according to O'Brien, the child died of lead poisoning. O'Brien warned that "personal cleanliness on the part of those handling lead or other poisons is not only a protection to themselves, but also to others, including their families." O'Brien's message to workers was clear: inattention to personal work habits hurts not just the worker but the worker's family as well.[1]

O'Brien's cautionary tale illustrates an important link between home and workplace, but it is in the form of a warning to workers and is aimed at changing their behavior. It also suggests that workers are capable of changing their personal environment, that is, their body and clothing, albeit with help from a new expert, the industrial hygienist. Significantly, O'Brien did not urge employers to change the workplace.

Industrial hygiene in the 1920s and 1930s evolved from modern science, professional and bureaucratic models, and the Progressive Era experience of protective labor laws. Larger environmental factors also influenced industrial hygiene, almost by necessity, because the worker's environment was the cause of many health problems. The influence of modern science made the dimensions of the workplace environment smaller, the targets more specific. Bureaucracies within newly formed state and federal labor departments created a number of areas of responsibility and expertise, one of which was industrial hygiene. Many of these new bureaucrats had been longtime activists for sex-based protective labor legislation.

This course was set in motion before World War I, when social reformers began to consider the industrial environment's reproductive hazards to women— as opposed to its socially damaging ones—but the growth of modern medicine, bureaucracies, and feminism in the 1920s influenced mainstream occupational health philosophies. For workers results were mixed. A healthy work environment was important, said reformers, because many women who worked in those environments were also mothers, and sick or poisoned workers could not raise children properly. But gender roles both contradicted and contributed to the ever narrower definitions of occupational disease that became current in the interwar years.[2] The relationship between home and workplace remained important, but industrial hygienists began to pay more attention to individual workers' behavior and, not unlike practitioners of what began to be called the "new public health," stressed the need for education. As science was accorded greater significance in workplace health and safety matters, employers became less likely to be blamed for illness. Placing the worker in a number of environments, each with its own hazards, theoretically diffused the responsibility for the causes of illness. Workers, not employers, would bear the responsibility for worker health.

Widening the wedge that had been created by the passage of female labor laws to provide protection for male workers gave reformers turned bureaucrats an opportunity to study women as workers, and not necessarily as mothers. Such reformer-bureaucrats understood that the work environment affected both men's and women's abilities to perform their jobs, and although the hazards to women were not always the same as to men, more often they were. For instance, Alice Hamilton felt compelled to connect the dangers of industrial lead poisoning to family members with a description of women workers who carried lead dust home in their hair; O'Brien knew that male workers risked harming their families with the same behavior. As a result many bureaucrats in state and federal women's and industrial hygiene agencies emphasized both gender sameness and gender difference in their studies.[3]

As we have seen, early proponents of female labor legislation had based their arguments on women's double duty and acknowledged that women's industrial working conditions affected their ability to be good mothers and homemakers. Consumers' Leagues reached this advocacy position through their middle-class sensibilities initially, not through firsthand knowledge of factory conditions. In the 1890s middle-class New York City matrons had begun to frequent the newly established department stores. As Susan Porter Benson has pointed out, working conditions in department stores were visible to the middle-class public in a way that factory conditions were not. Benson has accurately noted that the almost daily interaction between workers and customers in department stores affected far more middle-class women than that handful of factory inspectors who witnessed industrial conditions. Middle-class consumers observed for themselves that clerks remained on their feet for hours, often without rest periods or chairs. Holidays were most stressful, followed by the slack periods when clerks went without regular employment.[4]

The New York City Consumers' League, incorporated in 1891, initially appealed to the consciences of shoppers, urging them to shop early for Christmas in order not to overwork clerks. Members also drew up what they believed were fair working conditions, queried workers and managers regarding the degree to which their stores complied with Consumers' League standards, and then published a list of those retail stores with favorable, or at least adequate, conditions. They believed that consumers had a responsibility not only to avoid stores that treated their workers poorly but also to patronize actively those who did provide adequate wages, hours, and working conditions.[5]

The health of workers and the workplace more directly affected Consumers' League members' middle-class households when the league moved on to investigate industrial homework at the turn of the century. The manufacture of clothing, especially women's and children's clothing in tenement houses, provided a particularly striking example for the primarily female consumer public. It was not enough to appeal to consciences; self-interest also played a part. To middle-class women, seeing clothing made in filthy tenements raised the specter that they might themselves buy such unwholesome wares. Even though department store advertisers pointed out that it was easy to distinguish between tenement-shop garments and factory-made ones, diseased home workers posed a more serious problem. Many believed such workers could transmit germs from their bodies and environment to the garments they made.[6]

In an address before the New York City Consumers' League's 1904 annual meeting, Annie S. Daniel described accessories for women's dresses and hats being made "in the presence of small-pox" and children's and infant wear strewn on the beds of "children sick of contagious diseases." She warned members: "Into these little garments is sewed some of the contagion." Daniel, a physician at the New York Infirmary for Women and Children, pointed out that although consumers paid a little less for articles made in tenement houses, they risked being infected.[7]

Ten years later, the same league watched in dismay as manufacturers sent their tenement work across the river to New Jersey. But the Consumers' League of New Jersey soon picked up the trail and helped the Orange, New Jersey, Board of Health investigate "powder puffs" made by "little Italian children on the street curb." Investigators later found several of these puffs in the homes of polio victims.[8]

League members designed investigations of candy factories, also hot spots, to have a dramatic impact on the buying public. Reports of candy makers using spit-moistened fingers to separate paper candy cups, wearing dirty sweaters in

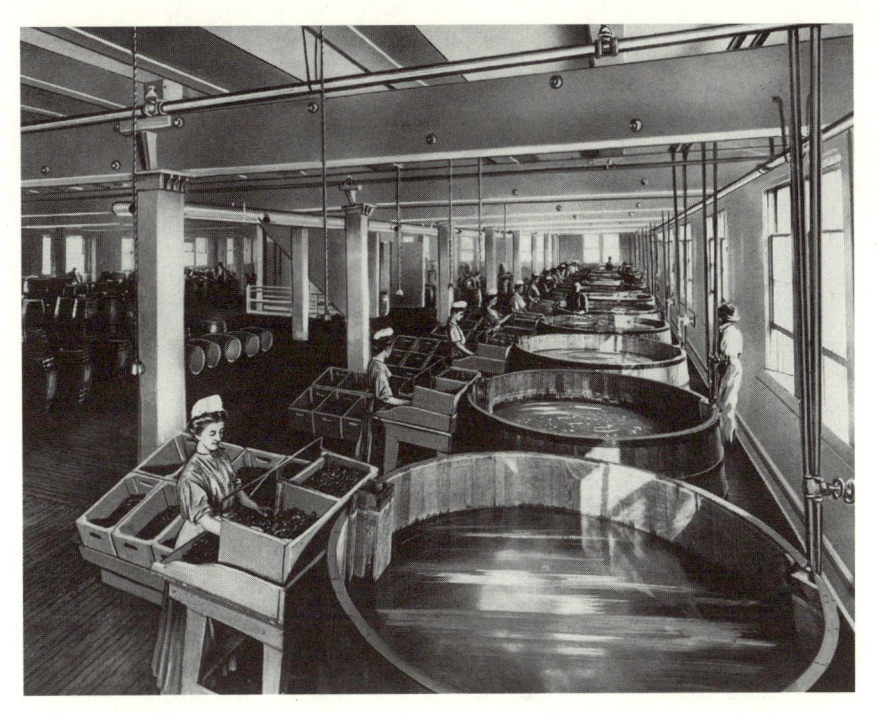

H.J. Heinz and Co. illustration of women sorting pickles, probably 1919. Women's Bureau notes point out the good lighting but also the lack of seating for workers.

the chilly dipping and packing rooms, and not having adequate washing facilities near toilets—all occurring amid sticky chocolate and sugar products—repelled a middle-class public imbued with modern notions of hygiene. At least one employer admitted that the public was indeed better off not knowing how candy was made.[9]

Employers responded in a variety of ways. According to the New York City Consumers' League president, Maud Nathan, some actively sought the Consumers' League stamp of approval—a "White List" in the retail trade and a "White Label" in the needle trades. Industries outside the league's self-defined jurisdiction encouraged investigations into their trades. While Nathan originally laughed at H.J. Heinz's proposal to apply Consumers' League standards to food processing, leagues in the Midwest and the West eventually used their influence to enforce hygiene and sanitation in the dairy industry.[10]

Other employers proudly publicized the conditions in which their female employees worked and provided descriptions that contrasted with those of the Consumers' League. Josephine Goldmark, in her 1912 study *Fatigue and Efficiency: A Study in Industry*, used the work of telephone operators as an example of the "new strain in industry." According to Goldmark the combination of "eleven separate processes" that each operator had to perform to complete one call, and the mental and physical exertion involved in keeping up with the large number and variety of calls, produced specific injuries to the operators' senses and nervous systems, as well as to their general health. In contrast, American Telephone and Telegraph emphasized the comfortable environment in which its operators worked, which included rest rooms complete with fireplaces and pianos, roof gardens, and hospital arrangements. Having already weeded out workers with less than ideal physical, mental, and moral qualifications, AT&T maintained that it did not overwork its operators. Managers instead described the complex series of telephone connections as a "game" where time passed quickly, with no sign of either monotony or overstrain.[11]

The Consumers' Leagues wanted to change the industrial environment, using as their strategy a depiction of the female worker as a victim of corporate greed. Leaguers took advantage of modern consumerism, aiming at the pocketbooks of both consumers and industry. They made explicit the ties between home and workplace by linking consumers' buying to working conditions and were successful in their appeal to consumers' fears about their own health, as opposed to purely humanitarian concerns about the worker. Publicly, however, the Consumers' League's national secretary, Florence Kelley, distinguished between means and ends, explaining to an audience in 1924 that the league did not seek to force retailers to reduce prices but to mobilize public opinion on behalf of "enlightened standards for workers and honest products for everybody." The leagues sought to achieve this through publicity about the poor health of women and children workers, which bred more disease, and against which the "purchaser of goods was defenseless."[12] Boycotts served two larger purposes—they forced a company to clean up and to make a "cleaner" product, and they theoretically created a better work environment for workers, the league's stated goal. Use of the boycott foreshadowed an environmentalist movement in the 1960s that also relied on linking workers and consumers.

Consumers' Leagues operated within an environmentalist worldview, one in which diseases caused by working conditions were easily transferred to private households. But the leagues went beyond earlier health reformers, who had stressed the connection between the worker and *her* home, and who believed that women's maternal responsibilities required healthy working conditions at the factory. Economic pressures brought by the Consumers' Leagues carried the environmentalist perspective into the middle-class household, potentially building a more solid case for protective labor legislation, as well as attempting to create cross-class gender solidarity. The leagues' success in awakening feelings of solidarity, however, was somewhat limited, since many members refused to submit

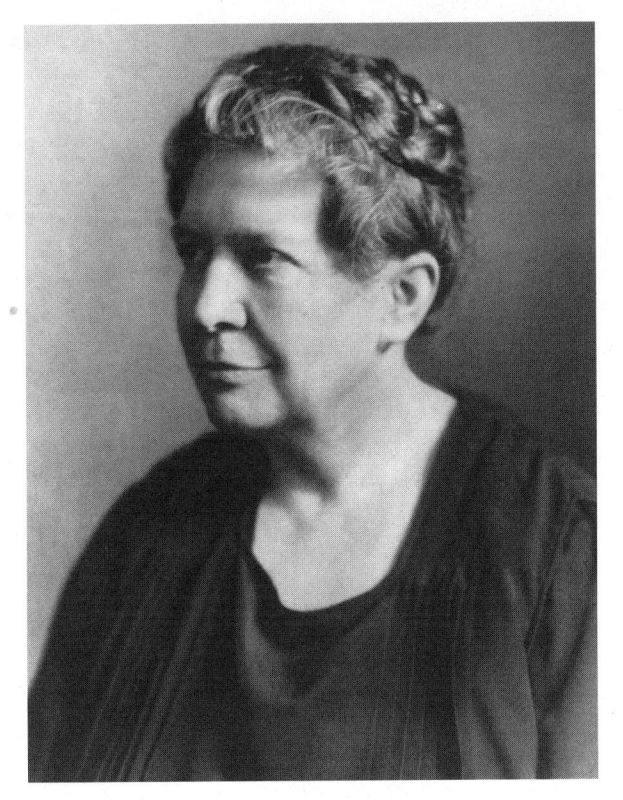

Florence Kelley, general secretary of the National Consumers' League.

domestic service and migrant farm labor to the scrutiny of state investigations. Beginning in the 1920s, Consumers' Leagues became vocal supporters of protective labor legislation, speaking against those who would have eliminated protective legislation through the passage of an Equal Rights Amendment.[13]

Debates over the ERA shaped gendered and non-gendered occupational health policies during this period, helping to initiate a shift in the definition of "environmentalism." Ironically, one of the major contributions of the Consumers' Leagues to this effort—the notion that a worker must be considered within his or her entire environment—became a tool by which workers became obliged to assume more responsibility for their own health, often deflecting responsibility from the employer.

The first debate on modern feminism, set in motion by the postsuffrage campaign for the Equal Rights Amendment in the 1920s, found its voice in the language of protective legislation. The ERA, a constitutional amendment introduced at every session of Congress since 1923, would mandate gender equality under the law. Pro-ERA forces argued that state protective laws restricting women's work hours kept women from being considered equal competitors in the paid workplace. Others believed protective laws were absolutely necessary for women whose wage work often occurred under unorganized, low-paying, and dirty conditions. State laws also recognized married women's double duty and presumably kept women from overwork.[14]

Popular images of the battle over the ERA in the 1920s have put women into two camps. At their most basic, these characterizations have placed one group in the position of opposing all laws that made distinctions between men and women, and the other group in the equally rigid position of promoting laws that perpetuated gender inequality. One group of feminists believed that an ERA would mandate gender equality in a way that suffrage did not and would also eliminate gender-based protective legislation, which was a glaring reminder that differences between men and women, not similarities, informed most workplace practices. The second group of feminists feared that eliminating protective legislation would irreparably damage the ability of working women to perform both their breadwinning tasks and their maternal duties. As Nancy Cott has shown, this dichotomy is too simplistic and ignores the complex web of gender, class, and politics that underscored postsuffrage feminism. Wendy Sarvasy has argued that the postsuffrage period not only presented more complications than previous historians have described but also, because of the sharp public division over the ERA, masked a common feminist agenda: gender equality within a construct of gender differentiation. In fact, real differences existed over the responsibility for health and the definition of "protection," but there was some agreement on other issues.[15]

ERA supporters correctly accused protectionists of viewing all women through one lens. Protectionists believed motherhood to be the primary role of all women, regardless of their current marital or maternal status. In some people's eyes, protecting women from their maternal instincts even provided the basis for these laws. They declared that a woman's nature would cause her to "throw aside every consideration . . . to nourish her young," often to the point of accepting low pay and risking her health. In contrast to working men, said one member of the Consumers' League of Connecticut, "There is not any kind of an old job in a factory that some woman will not do" to provide for her children. The workplace environment, therefore, was critical to the health of society's mothers, and protectionists believed that that link mandated the protection of all women through prescribing shorter hours. Gender-based labor legislation painted all women with the same broad brush and often ignored women's individual work needs. Those who supported an ERA believed that they considered women as individuals, each capable of looking after her own interests. Women's health needs were best addressed by providing women with all the economic, educational, and political opportunities available to men.[16]

Arguments on both sides influenced occupational health, but in different ways. First, protectionists in large part became bureaucrats in state and federal women's bureaus, urging the extension of female labor laws limiting hours and night work and establishing minimum wages. These bureaucrats institutionalized gender-based workplace policies, but they also advocated better protection for all workers through hours legislation and workers' compensation coverage for occupational disease. By the 1920s many states had established women's bureaus, usually within the state departments of labor and usually oriented around the problems of women in industry. Female reformers involved in the New York State Factory Investigating Commission and the Women's Trade Union League in the 1910s, including Frances Perkins, Nelle Swartz, and Frieda Miller, joined the state's Department of Labor in the 1920s and 1930s. Using health as the main criterion, they found themselves in a good position to lobby for legislation for women.[17]

In 1926 the New York State industrial commissioner, relying on information from the Bureau of the Division of Women in Industry, supported the Forty-Eight Hour Law for women because he agreed that health considerations were of first importance both for the mother and the next generation. When the commissioner argued that modern industrialism created strain and prevented adequate rest and recreation, he acknowledged the close interaction between home and work that had so impressed the Factory Investigating Commission team. Even without the status of formal elective or appointive position, women reformers like Eleanor Roosevelt, long active in the Women's Trade Union League, used their positions within the state Democratic Party to argue in favor of the Forty-Eight Hour Law.[18]

In 1924, in *Radice v. The People of the State of New York,* the U.S. Supreme Court had shown its willingness to prohibit night work for women, a decision praised at the time by the industrial commissioner, Bernard Shientag. In making its decision, the Court had relied on the evidence collected by the Factory Investigating Commission and the advocacy of the Bureau of Women in Industry to determine that night work created conditions "detrimental to the health of women." It was difficult enough for anyone to obtain a restful night's sleep during the day, said the Court, but this was particularly so for women, who had more delicate constitutions, as well as daytime functions peculiar to their sex, namely housework.[19]

Minimum wage legislation often went hand in hand with protective labor laws; support for it, too, was rooted in concern for women's health. The New

York State Bureau of Women in Industry noted a relationship between poverty and ill health and believed that "starvation wages" made it impossible for women to "maintain themselves in health and to supply the very necessaries of life." The 1937 State Minimum Wage Law required wage boards to consider the cost of maintaining an adequate lifestyle for women, including sufficient income for medical care. Statewide financial data were used to argue that clothing and food budgets were also essential for good health. The bureau's understanding of health continued to indicate the importance of the relationship between home and work, something construed quite differently for male workers. Labor unions often bargained for higher wages for men based on the idea of a "family wage" sufficient to provide for the whole family and to keep workers' wives out of the paid workforce entirely.[20]

Reformers also gained a national audience. With the 1920 creation of the Women's Bureau of the U.S. Department of Labor, the protectionist feminists who comprised much of the bureau's staff had more access to resources and the potential for making a bigger difference.[21] The Women's Bureau became a strong advocate of shorter hours and better sanitary conditions for working women throughout the 1920s and 1930s. During this period it accepted both the primacy of science and the protection of motherhood. Its emphasis on working women's economic imperatives led to an agenda that recognized both the factory and the household workloads of women. The bureau issued a number of bulletins in 1921; many of these reflected its reliance on scientific authority. It called for the "scientific study of the effect on [women's] health, and that of future generations, of exploitation, long hours, and improper working conditions." To reduce the deleterious effects on women of lifting heavy weights on the job, the bureau also supported scientific management theories that analyzed the careful coordination of human muscles. Such studies were to be conducted by new professionals—scientists and health experts as well as industrial engineers.[22]

Using a rationale similar to that put forth by other supporters of shorter workdays for women, the Women's Bureau acknowledged that working women's maternal and household responsibilities affected their workplace health and performance. Women as mothers deserved to be protected because they were mothers, and women workers found that the extra burden of motherhood sometimes adversely affected their job performance. Thus, the Women's Bureau found itself arguing for better workplace conditions in order to preserve the health of women, which, in turn, created better home conditions for themselves and their families.

The Women's Bureau also acknowledged that the nonindustrial environment affected the workplace. Poverty, for instance, created physical conditions that impaired women's ability to be effective at a strenuous job. In this conclusion the bureau had the support of many women physicians. Drawing parallels to public fears about women physicians' health a generation earlier, Rosalie Slaughter-Morton admitted that working-class women have "always had to work pretty hard." This alumna of Woman's Medical College in Philadelphia believed that opposition to working women came from an overestimation of the "pelvis and its contents" and an underestimation of the rest of the body. With a pointed reference to working-class poverty, Slaughter-Morton suggested that some working women were frail not because they worked but because they suffered from malnutrition and unhealthy living conditions. In such cases, she went on, women may find better conditions at work—regular hours, camaraderie, a positive if impersonal approach to work, not to mention regular income—than they could find at home.[23]

The ERA also had an influence on occupational health. Women's Bureau investigators who resented being accused by the most public pro-ERA organization of the period, the National Woman's Party, of opposing equal rights, were sensitive to the party's charge that the Women's Bureau considered women inferior. Throughout the 1920s and 1930s, the bureau's investigators were careful to avoid antagonizing the party. In 1934, for example, the bureau's director, Mary Anderson, decided against trying to include special guidelines for women in one of the National Recovery Act Codes because she was reluctant to get into an argument with the National Woman's Party.[24]

Ultimately the Women's Bureau advocated healthier and safer workplace conditions for all workers. Its research on women's exposure to nonreproductive occupational diseases had industry-wide implications, since many of these conditions also affected men. The bureau wanted to eliminate hazards for women not by prohibiting women from dangerous jobs but by cleaning up the workplace. "Prohibiting the employment of women on certain dusty processes," wrote one investigator, "does not solve the problem of any industrial disease in a community." Like many in the bureau, this writer recognized the inconsistencies inherent in restricting women from working conditions they had long faced at home. She feared that it was "very possible that under the guise of 'protection' women may be shut out from occupations which are really less harmful to them than much of the tedious heavy work both in the home and in the factory which has long been considered their special province."[25]

Women workers themselves, especially the growing number of married workers, balanced the often conflicting priorities of unpaid housework and paid wage work outside the home. Laundry workers, department store clerks, and factory hands all recognized the impact of workplace conditions on their living situation and acted to strike the best compromise, whether it was to support (or oppose) night work restrictions or perhaps to consider the advantages of

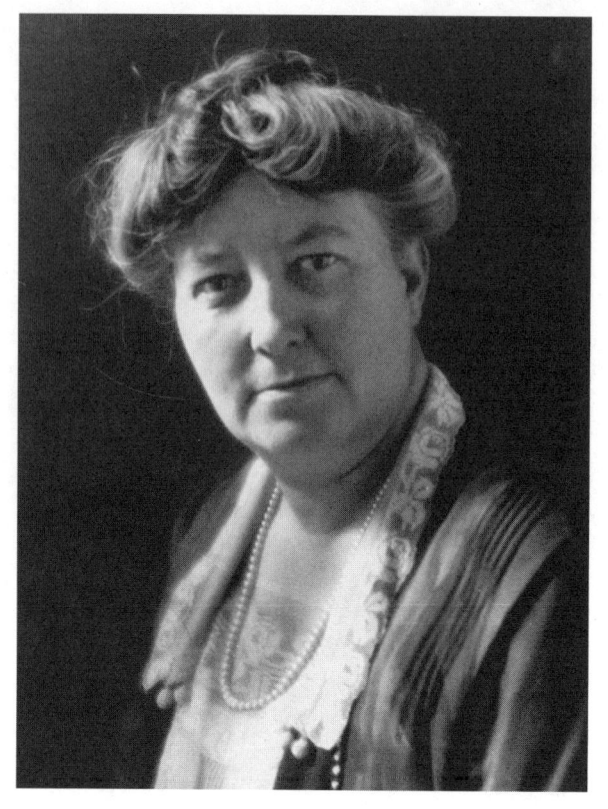

Mary Anderson, first director, Women's Bureau of the U.S. Department of Labor.

homework. For example, despite the National Consumers' League's characterization of night work as detrimental to all women, some married women clearly preferred it because it often allowed them to avoid child care problems, especially if their husbands worked days. Similar rationales underlay some working-class women's support for tenement work.[26]

Ideas about women's protection and equality were not the only influence on workplace health. Changes in medicine, especially its role in industry and in government, also contributed to the narrower conception of industrial health. First came industrial physicians. From its tentative introduction at the turn of the century in mining and lumber industries and in urban hospitals, industrial medicine by 1921 was devoted more to keeping workers on the job and less to uncovering new occupational diseases, although industrial physicians claimed responsibility for detecting new ways of protecting workers from the diseases that did exist.[27]

Alice Hamilton was underwhelmed at the ability of some company physicians to detect known hazards like lead poisoning. When she conducted a series of investigations in Ohio, she encountered a physician at a pottery plant who had treated several women for "hysterical convulsions" but who had never thought to ask his patients if they worked with lead glaze. She also worried about the objectivity of company physicians, noting that although physicians at the National Lead Company smelting plant had reported four cases of lead poisoning during a six-month period, she found 105 in just twice that time.[28]

With little time spent in clinical and laboratory research, industrial physicians nevertheless fashioned a specialty that influenced the direction of occupational health for both women and men workers. While defining their medical jurisdiction broadly, industrial physicians helped construe occupational health ever more narrowly. They believed that the risks posed by industrial disease paled in comparison to the great variety of non-occupational ills that workers exposed themselves to in the sixteen hours they were not at their trade. Praising the work of Hamilton and others at Harvard University's School of Public Health, Harold Stevens, the medical director of Jordan Marsh department store, told Boston-area physicians that the "group of special industrial diseases, relatively small, [was] growing smaller in fact of incidence as knowledge of environmental control [was] extended." The industrial physician's value to public health, then, lay in educating workers and changing their personal behavior and habits. Industrial physicians, according to Christopher Sellers, looked to the body rather than the environment for answers.[29]

Industrial physicians emphasized the need to treat workers as more than just workers and to be aware of the other aspects of their lives, but they tended to blame conditions other than those of the plant to explain illness. When Stevens posed the question, "Is industrial management responsible for all the ills of an industrial society?" he presumed the answer to be no. It is important to remember, however, that industrial physicians were themselves employees. In any event, industrial medicine's understanding of environmentalism, which minimized the significance of the workplace in favor of the non-occupational world, contrasted sharply with the environmentalism of reformers like the National Consumers' League.[30]

Historians have studied changes in public health campaigns during this period. Known as the "new public health," these policies were rooted in germ theory and focused on education and prevention rather than on broad environmental solutions to public health. As a result, according to Richard A. Meckel, public health professionals who worried about infant mortality rates, for instance, shared industrial physicians' beliefs that targeting individual behavior would create a healthier and more efficient society. Even Hamilton, writing in 1916, had acknowledged the importance of distinguishing between "general cleanliness" and "specific protection against infection" and had urged individual vigilance against disease. Her attitude, however, was mediated by her strong social concerns.[31]

The interaction of modern medicine with modern industry led many hygienists to focus on the specific, and this orientation stands in sharp contrast to that of the Women's Bureau. Hygienists looked at physiological changes in order to pinpoint disease. As industrial hygienists and industrial physicians sought to create a body of expert knowledge that they would control, they viewed themselves as the gatekeepers of knowledge about industrial hygiene which they alone would pass on to the worker. Emphases on bacteriology and chemistry also led hygienists to attribute disease to individual behaviors, such as the lack of attention to personal hygiene. Illness became the result of workers' own failings. Like public health officials during this period, hygienists emphasized individual responsibility. Research compiled by the Illinois Division of Industrial Hygiene on radium poisoning prompted hygienists to write at length about the need to hire only workers with good hygiene and work habits and to avoid applicants who bit their nails, refused to wear proper head coverings, or did not wash their hands thoroughly. Avoidance of radium poisoning, to them, lay more in changing personal habits than in changing workplace conditions.[32]

The hygienists' brand of environmentalism added complexity to industrial hygiene. Many hygienists viewed the worker primarily as a citizen, with a variety of activities and influences outside the workplace—some of which affected the job. In treating the "whole worker," hygienists and industrial physicians felt they first needed to understand the variety of "bodily processes," both physiological and chemical, of each worker, noting that changes in any of these might affect response to long-term exposure to certain workplace hazards.[33]

Moreover, some doctors believed that such common complaints as colds, headaches, or dysmenorrhea could be reduced by attention to workplace factors that contributed to these ailments. One hygienist argued that such complaints might be warning signs of "low resistance and excessive fatigue." In any event diagnosis was complex, they argued, because of the multiplicity of symptoms that might be either normal or indicative of occupational exposure, depending on the person's individual makeup.[34]

In this intellectual climate more emphasis was inevitably given to diagnostic techniques. For example, the definition of what constituted lead poisoning changed during this period. In the aftermath of a well-publicized tetra-ethyl lead incident in 1924–1925, where five male workers died of acute lead poisoning, and forty-nine were seriously poisoned as a result of the introduction of lead into gasoline, hygienists and academics focused on establishing threshold-limit values under which workers would be considered "safe" from acute lead poisoning.[35] Chronic lead poisoning, however, had always been more problematic for workers, physicians, and employers, albeit for different reasons. Workers sought adequate protection from a condition that occurred almost silently over a long period of time. Physicians found the ways in which lead was detected, excreted, and stored in the body intriguing. And employers wanted to limit the number of cases of lead poisoning, especially if it constituted a compensable industrial disease. One way to do that involved examining more carefully the process by which poisoning occurred.

A lead line along the gums of workers had long been an indication of exposure to lead but, by the early 1930s, that line was harder to find, thanks to better dental hygiene. At a February 1931 meeting of the Massachusetts Medico-Legal Society, Hamilton distinguished between actual absorption and exposure. Finding lead in workers' urine and stool did not, by itself, indicate absorption, explained Hamilton, because lead could be excreted without being absorbed. She believed that blood tests showing "stippled red cells" provided the most accurate diagnosis, although she preferred to see the presence of a variety of other symptoms and test results before diagnosing lead poisoning.[36]

May Mayers agreed with her. As a physician for the New York State Bureau of Industrial Hygiene, Mayers had been trying to define lead poisoning since 1926, after it became a compensable disease under New York State law. In the 1930s she worked to develop a series of criteria with both clinical and laboratory signs of lead poisoning, from physical symptoms in the gastrointestinal tract, the nervous system, or the musculoskeletal structure, to blood, urine, or stool changes. No single indication or symptom would be enough to diagnose poisoning. In fact clinical symptoms acted only as the starting point for a variety of laboratory tests. Mayers consistently argued that individual susceptibility determined lead absorption, which would be detected on a case-by-case basis: "The quantity of lead which may be present in the circulation at a given time without producing toxic effects is largely a matter of personal idiosyncracy."[37]

Industry preferred this approach. If lead poisoning had to meet a number of different tests, then fewer cases would be diagnosed. The lead industry had long charged an overabundance of misdiagnoses from industrial hygienists and general practitioners. Companies who used lead also frequently pointed out the amount of lead already normally found in "modern civilized communities." While industry officials agreed with Mayers about the need for multiple signs of poisoning, they disagreed over which signs to accept. Mayers believed that lead poisoning was indicated by any sign of lead found in blood, urine, or stool samples, regardless of clinical symptoms. Industry representatives, including Robert Kehoe of the Charles F. Kettering Laboratory, believed that the body could absorb and excrete a varying amount of lead without being poisoned. Both, however, agreed that if the worker was not suffering, there was no poisoning.[38]

The increasingly specific diagnosis developed for lead poisoning had its effect on women workers. In the 1920s Mayers wrote that women were more susceptible to lead poisoning and should therefore be prohibited from working with the metal. By 1938 she had refined her concerns about women and lead. Evidence suggested that children of both mothers and fathers who worked with lead seemed adversely affected by their parents' exposure. There seems to have been no laboratory test for men or women, however, for testing reproductive changes due to the presence of lead, and evidence continued to be based on symptoms reported by workers. In the meantime industry officials produced results of laboratory tests on animals showing no fertility problems in the presence of lead, even though lead did show up in the placentas of pregnant rats and the milk of lactating ones. By the late 1930s a number of diagnostic devices became available to test for lead poisoning, which was defined as meeting a specific set of clinical and laboratory standards. With respect to reproductive hazards, dangers to both men and women were recognized, but neither the National Safety Council nor Mayers was willing to prohibit all women from working with lead, only pregnant and lactating women.[39]

The increased specificity of diagnosis of industrial disease seems to have promised working women more choices—or at least placed in their hands the ability to make some choices for themselves. Not only did a variety of concerned parties express relatively less interest in protecting women's social roles in the household as mothers, but in the years just prior to World War II, they also appeared less concerned about protecting women's biological, maternal abilities.

Some physicians used women workers for research on women. When medical diagnosis became more highly targeted, much of the research on working women shifted away from studies of the ill effects of industrial work and toward investigations of working women as women rather than as women workers. The Massachusetts epidemiologist Mary Lakeman studied menstrual pain in 365 industrial women in 1933. Lakeman found that 89.6 percent of women reported some kind of pain during their periods. Noting no significant differences between women who did different types of work, Lakeman instead surmised that class might be a better indicator of dysmenorrhea. She cited a similar study of college-educated women that showed far fewer self-reported cases of menstrual pain. Although she believed it was possible that working-class women actually suffered more due to an "inactive" lifestyle, Lakeman put more credence in both cultural and psychological differences: college women had an "improved attitude" about menstruation and a more "independent" lifestyle, which presumably led to fewer days off due to dysmenorrhea. In contrast, working-class women respondents might have been exhibiting a "cultural attitude of invalidism," which Lakeman found prevalent in the working class. It could be, wrote Lakeman, that "working girls take every opportunity to take off sick."[40]

Although it seems clear that Lakeman, a physician, spoke from a favorable socioeconomic position, her attitudes are worth examining in the context of occupational health. On the one hand, her willingness to attribute menstrual pain to broader cultural circumstances may be seen as acknowledging a cause-and-effect relationship between environment and health. Indeed, many physicians had begun to pay attention to the psychological aspects of menstruation. On the other hand, her reluctance to consider alternative explanations or even to question the validity of her results illustrates an increasingly common scenario that stressed the social environment over the workplace as the origin of ill health.[41]

What did all this mean for workers? First, the meaning of "environment" changed. More distance was placed between workers and their workplace environment even as former reformers brought the industrial workplace closer to the home. Increased diagnostic precision refined the boundaries of what constituted health and disease. Efforts to widen the jurisdiction of industrial physicians diluted the number of workplace-caused illnesses. And emphasis on individual characteristics placed more responsibility on individuals to maintain health. Finally, treating women as workers sometimes resulted in the establishment of standards for all workers based on the behavior of women workers.

By connecting health to industrial efficiency, Josephine Goldmark had tried to convince employers that it was in their best interests to do what was necessary to keep women workers safe for their home responsibilities. By the 1930s a significant reversal had occurred. Efficiency experts tried to maintain a proper, that is, efficient, workplace by changing not the industrial but the nonindustrial environment. The private household was no longer an unchanging sphere of maternal activity that needed to be preserved and protected. It became a place that could and should be manipulated to achieve industrial efficiency. By obtaining more public roles for women, industry adopted both the language of protectionists and the ideology of ERA supporters. But it used these to attempt the social control of workers in this period.

Protectionists turned bureaucrats did, however, manage to bring the language of domesticity into the workplace, informed by their understanding that working women's health easily traversed the boundaries of home and factory. Not unlike female urban reformers twenty years earlier, industrial hygienists in New York urged employers to pay attention to "industrial housekeeping" by reducing the fumes and dusts that often permeated the workplace.[42] Sharing industrial physicians' interest in the detection and control of toxicity in new chemicals, New York State industrial hygienists like Mayers, Adelaide Ross-Smith, and, later, Olive Kooyman, also urged workers to pay attention to personal hygiene. A cleaner workplace represented a safe and healthy workplace—not unlike the home.[43]

Applying household skills to the workplace implies that it is an environment that can be kept clean by relatively simple means. Two before-and-after photographs of a workbench, one in disarray and one very tidy, graced the pages of a 1920s *Industrial Hygiene Bulletin*. In contrast to previous efforts by reformers to link home and workplace in order to attract attention to workplace hazards, hygienists now used the imagery of the private household to describe the ideal industrial environment. Such imagery also served to de-emphasize the dangers of the workplace.

Employers borrowed environmentalism as understood by protectionists to shift responsibility for illness to any number of causes other than the workplace. In the pursuit of "health" for workers, they also provided a variety of on-the-job medical services. Despite many employers' reluctance to provide broad-ranging health care to their workers, industrial nurses and physicians performed a variety of duties, sometimes visiting the workers' homes, providing child care, and performing other nonmedical services. Early diagnosis and treatment, argued one medical officer in a department store, benefited both the company and the employer, and avoided having the worker need to visit the family physician or the hospital.[44]

The interest that employers took in keeping workers on the job can be traced to their obligation to pay for injuries incurred at work regardless of fault. Not surprisingly, many companies with medical services employed a nurse to follow up on sick or injured workers, not only making sure that workers were not just loafing but also observing personal habits that could affect job performance. As a representative of Walworth Manufacturing in Massachusetts explained to his colleagues in the Manufacturers' Research Association, the visiting nurse he employed would help an ill worker "if there is a good reason for his being out," but if not, "he will have to change his habits if he is to remain in our employ."[45]

A worker's individual makeup and reaction to a specific hazard prompted greater emphasis on individual characteristics rather than group norms. While pro-ERA feminists promoted this focus on the individual as a means to advance the position of women in the workplace, it had the effect of diverting responsibility from the hazards of the workplace, a diversion that helped neither female nor male workers. Taking advantage of the weak position of organized labor during this period, a series of radio messages entitled "Health in Industry" began airing in Massachusetts in 1931. These messages, sponsored and prepared by the Massachusetts Medical Society's Committee on Public Education for the

State Department of Public Health, placed the responsibility for health squarely on workers. Commenting on the higher sickness rate of women workers, the radio announcer accused women of not understanding the relationship between health and individual achievement. He went on to predict that during this period of high unemployment, the most physically fit would get the available jobs. Nearly seven months later, another broadcast emphasized that good health was an individual concern. It must be made clear to workers, intoned the announcer, that "sickness is largely the individual's own responsibility."[46]

Many industrial physicians determined physical fitness through pre-employment and pre-placement physical examinations. With the passage of workers' compensation statutes, it made economic sense for employers to scrutinize carefully applicants who had respiratory problems, for instance, before employing them in a dusty workplace. Universal Winding Company in Massachusetts checked employees for hernias before assigning them to the foundry or other heavy lifting jobs. Employers also wanted physicians to look for such physical defects as poor eyesight or hearing.[47]

Workers, physicians, feminists, and employers responded differently to these examinations. Workers correctly suspected that such exams were used to exclude those with marginal defects or even those with radical tendencies. For their part industrial physicians believed that careful examinations placed workers in "jobs appropriate to their physical conditions," according to Christopher Sellers. Exams also alerted physicians to non-occupational medical problems, which they often treated in the interests of reducing lost time. The presence of in-plant dispensaries tended to reduce company insurance rates. Members of the National Woman's Party applauded increased use of physical examinations for workers because they believed that the consideration of individual rather than group physical characteristics would improve women's chances at better job opportunities. "Natural fitness," argued Doris Stevens, would separate some women from all women and, she implied, some women from some men.[48]

Economics rather than occupational health concerns drove manufacturers. The Manufacturers' Research Association, formed by a group of Boston-area business owners in 1925, regularly inspected one anothers' factories or manufacturing plants, recorded observations, and made recommendations for greater efficiency, quality, and health and safety. Managers repeatedly noted when jobs performed by men could just as easily be performed by women for less money. Their interest in health and safety lay in reducing accidents from faulty machine guards, tripping hazards, and other non-gendered issues. When observations about dust hazards surfaced, respondents usually explained them in one of two ways, both of which illustrate the influence of increased specificity: either

(1) "vegetable dusts" such as those produced by cotton were not dangerous; or (2) workers did not wear the respirators provided by the company.

New England textile manufacturers openly criticized maximum weekly hours laws for women—fifty-four in Maine, New Hampshire, and Rhode Island, fifty-five in Connecticut, and forty-eight in Massachusetts—not because they supported equal rights for women, but because of the competitive edge they lost to southern mills, which operated under no such restrictions. Since textile manufacturers employed large numbers of women, owners thought it impractical to run their mills beyond the weekly limit that women could legally work, even though this decision resulted in a "considerable Southern advantage in its ability to make machinery and equipment more productive." The Women's Bureau dismissed their complaints, alleging increased productivity in textile plants after the passage of the Forty-Eight Hour Law in Massachusetts. According to its research, re-needlers threaded 32,000 needles a day during fifty-four-hour weeks, but clocked 39,000 to 41,000 per day when they worked forty-eight hours a week. New England physicians applauded the Women's Bureau's sentiment regarding the need to protect womanhood but believed it resulted in a competitive disadvantage to Massachusetts textile mills, and instead tried to promote Massachusetts as a responsible example to other states.[49]

In some cases, gendered interest in workplace conditions resulted the extension of standards originally established for women to male workers. In the 1930s a Harvard Business School researcher, Elton Mayo, studied a group of women at Western Electric's Hawthorne Plant in Chicago. After implementing a series of changes in the workplace that sought to test (and eventually improve) productivity, Mayo determined that women workers who assembled relays not only responded favorably to rest periods and shorter workdays, they also performed more efficiently when they had amenable and informal social interaction. In other words, they responded positively to noneconomic factors in the workplace. The "Hawthorne Effect"—the existence of unexpected influences of nonexperimental variables—became a tool that personnel managers continue to use to influence the behavior and productivity of thousands of workers, male and female.[50]

Mayo wanted to quantify fatigue. He conducted detailed interviews and numerous work experiments with a group of six women and made several unsuccessful attempts to link a wide range of variables, including menstruation, to poor work performance. Researchers questioned these women regularly about their home and social lives, and the women visited the company hospital once a month. Researchers who tried to understand changes in work performance looked not at working conditions but instead sought some measurable physiological change caused by non-occupational factors—futilely, as it turned out.[51]

In the beginning of the century, female reformers who worried about the effects of overwork on women workers had viewed fatigue with concern and had advocated rest periods. This provided employers with a model for male workers. Alan Derickson has described the introduction of short rest periods in the 1910s among women workers. Male workers at first refused to accept such practices, characterizing them as "effeminate," although they eventually changed their minds. A common thread runs through this research, that of studying the physiological and psychological effects of fatigue on women. The goals, however, differed. Josephine Goldmark wanted to change occupational factors to reduce fatigue; Mayo sought to discover which non-occupational habits tired women.[52]

Not all professionals and bureaucrats wanted to change the worker. The Women's Bureau refused to blame the victim. It consistently placed responsibility for cleaning up the workplace on state government and industry. The bureau preferred workers' compensation laws that covered occupational diseases and mandatory reporting, which would protect men and women. "When industry must pay for the diseases it produces," wrote Margaret Mettert, "better processes of handling and production will result."[53]

The bureau also continued to pay attention to hazards common to women who worked in largely female-dominated industries. Women most frequently reported dermatitis, which accounted for from 60 percent to nearly 87 percent of all cases in a five-state survey in the 1930s. Cleaning agents, dyes, certain fruits and vegetables, oils and greases, rubber, plastics, and mica all contained skin irritants that produced mild or more serious infections. During World War I and World War II, the bureau added tetryl and fulminate of mercury to the list. Women in manufacturing, domestic service, and sales jobs—the last two primarily performed by women—reported cases of synovitis (an inflammation of the wrist) and other diseases resulting from repetitive activity, such as those used in gripping or pulling motions and in the continuous use of hand tools. In addition, exposure to mica, silica, and clay dust produced respiratory diseases like pneumoconiosis.[54]

Like the bureau, Hamilton, although part of the government and of academia by the 1920s, did not give up her ties to broad grassroots reformism. Evidence for this is her vice presidency of the National Consumers' League for more than twenty years and her continued part-time residence at Hull House. Hamilton tried hard to retain what Paul Kellogg called a "real human setting" in her articles about industrial disease. Kellogg, editor of the muckraking magazines *The Survey* and *The Survey Graphic,* reminded Hamilton of her moral obligation to the magazine's "socially minded audience," even as he recognized that the world of industrial hygiene was changing. He lamented to Hamilton in

1923 that, twenty years ago, "You could take up industrial accidents by telling of their bloody and preventable occurrences. Today the real issue hinges around some point in compensation law." Nevertheless, Hamilton's 1924 article on the hatting industry, "A Medieval Industry in the Twentieth Century" for *The Survey* managed to scrape together enough danger to elicit critical comment from hat manufacturers.[55]

The influences of feminism and of industrial medicine resulted in scientific studies on workers and workplaces in the interwar years that emphasized individual differences to match the employee to the work, as well as technology that would eliminate all industrial accidents except those due to worker error. These influences had equally mixed results for men and women. But sometimes gains for women as workers did not translate into gains for all workers.

4

Women in Wartime Industries: "We Want Steel Toes like the Men"

Alma worked the night shift in 1943 in order to have her days free for the house and kids. She slept about five or six hours a day, never all at one time. Irregular heat and ventilation in the plant where she worked and the cold she caught there left her with a cough, but she did not go home sick. When her husband and kids caught cold, however, she stayed out of work for a week to nurse them. Still, Alma found the work preferable to full-time housewifery and wanted to continue it after the war, somehow balancing it with her family and household responsibilities.[1]

The *New York Times* writer Elizabeth Hawes used Alma's story to illustrate why absenteeism was high among working mothers during World War II. Alma's experience also suggests two important and contradictory aspects of the war with respect to occupational health. First, Alma asked no special favors at work, suffering the same discomfort as other workers, both male and female. She expected to be accorded both the freedom and the responsibility to make employment decisions for herself. Second, the reality of Alma's household responsibilities, even with a caring husband who pitched in with meals for the kids and dishwashing, meant that her family's health was directly tied to hers, which in turn affected how she interacted with the workplace.[2]

Many wage-earning women expected equal treatment and equal protection but also knew that domestic responsibilities influenced women's workplace performance. This was the dual nature of the wartime workplace, and it revealed the tensions built into feminist notions of equality and special treatment. The war brought the trade-offs and contradictions inherent in these tensions into sharp focus, allowing employers to limit occupational health and safety changes and women workers to incorporate these trade-offs into the reality of their lives.

For instance, feminist activism for sex equality coincided with employers' priorities of achieving full wartime production with minimal changes to accommodate women. Equal treatment was also championed by many women workers who sought expanded economic opportunities. This was in conflict with another perspective, that of gender difference, especially the double duty that distinguished female workers from their male counterparts. The experience of World War II reveals that women workers and employers alike believed that, in the short term, occupational health should be focused more on reducing gender distinctions than on changing the workplace environment or its boundaries. In the long, postwar term, however, heightened fears about reproductive hazards prompted employers to reconsider the significance of gender difference. Women workers who were excluded from jobs with reproductive hazards realized that changes in the workplace environment were essential to full equality and a healthy home life.

War-related industries in the United States mobilized when Europe went to war in 1939. Industries recruiting women increased greatly after the United States entered the conflict in December 1941. Within six months employers had increased their estimates of the proportion of new jobs available to women from 29 percent to 55 percent. The War Manpower Commissioner, Paul V. McNutt, asserted that women were capable of performing 80 percent of war jobs. By 1944, 16 percent of wage-earning women were working in such war-related industries as aircraft, shipbuilding, and munitions. In most cases this constituted a dramatic increase; females accounted for only 5 percent of auto workers in April 1942 but about 25 percent eighteen months later.[3]

Public pronouncements about the war exhorted women to do their duty to defeat Hitler, to be the "soldierettes" of the home front by doing the work needed to build war matériel, regardless of potential dangers or "unfemininess." In contrast to earlier efforts to keep women away from adverse working conditions, employment managers during World War II clearly expected more from women. "Women should be told what to expect," declared a Tennessee supervisor. They should not be allowed to quit or be absent because of dirty, noisy, wet, dusty, or poorly ventilated conditions. The War Manpower Commission de-emphasized physical differences between men and women and pointed to European women, particularly Germans, who successfully performed "an almost limitless number of jobs, many of which require[d] considerable physical exertion." Appeals to patriotism went hand in hand with warnings about the unsuitability of certain jobs for most women, most frequently those requiring heavy lifting. Citing Women's Bureau statistics rating the "average woman's" strength at 570/1000 of a man's and her physical resistance at 697/1000, public officials initially urged employers to avoid hiring women for jobs that risked coercing them to exceed their strength.[4]

Several informal and formal policies governed hiring practices. Employers were restricted by custom, as the sex segregation of the industrial workplace had long limited the types of jobs available to women. Not until large numbers of men began leaving for military duty did defense-related industries begin to hire

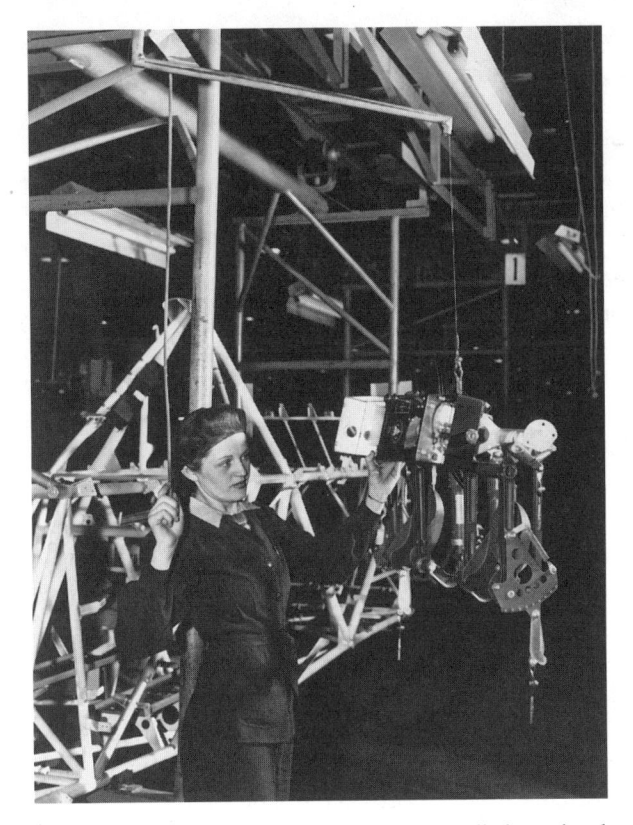

Vultee Aircraft Company in California installed overhead cranes during World War II to enable women workers to lift assemblies that weighed more than the 25-pound state limit. Many companies found that such engineering changes also appealed to male workers.

women in significant numbers.[5] Where workplace health was concerned, employers followed the regulations that originated with state labor and health departments. Factory inspections had long subjected employers to state scrutiny, establishing safety standards in many workplaces, and workers' compensation insurance provided injured workers with a state-mandated, employer-financed disability benefit. By the beginning of the war many states also carried compensation insurance for at least some occupational diseases that resulted in disability. Although benefits went only to workers who became disabled, the threat of higher premiums for accident-prone enterprises presumably nudged employers to employ preventive health and safety measures in the workplace. Workers' compensation covered both male and female workers.[6]

Employers had to work within the boundaries of protective laws aimed at women only. Protective legislation reflected a number of assumptions that highlighted sex and gender differences. The Women's Bureau believed that women's primary social responsibilities lay in their qualities as caretakers of house and children and feared that wage-earning women, urged by employers, would, without legislation, work so many hours in the factory that they would be too run down to perform household duties properly.[7] Supporters of a national Equal Rights Amendment, including the National Woman's Party, however, had long believed that an individual approach to industrial health and safety, not blanket protective laws, would best advance women's position in the workforce.

The influx of larger numbers of women into the industrial workplace by 1942 presented very real logistical problems for employers who sought to reconcile protective legislation with wartime production goals. When a Buffalo, New York, machine-gun bullet manufacturer with a largely female labor force initially expanded production from one to three shifts to accommodate wartime demand, it had to hire men for the evening and night shifts because New York labor laws prohibited women from working between 10 P.M. and 6 A.M. But men proved "unable to adapt themselves to the work" and were much less efficient, according to the general manager, Edmund W. Walker, and the company was compelled to institute longer day shifts, "so that we needed to hire only girls." Many states agreed to a temporary lifting of sex-based protective labor laws or at least gave employers an opportunity to apply for exceptions. Employers promised to ease restrictions in the name of "common sacrifice" only for the duration of the war.[8]

But workplace hazards had by no means been eliminated. To the contrary, the expansion of production increased the likelihood of injury or illness. The introduction of new materials and processes, the larger proportion of unskilled workers, and greater exposure to existing chemical hazards because of longer hours all made the workplace more dangerous. Nevertheless, both employers and newly hired women hoped to keep accidents or illness to a minimum. For employers that meant treating women workers as much like men as possible, including an emphasis on personal responsibility for health and safety and the re-engineering of some workplace sites. Some practical, specific responses to the physical workplace accommodated women's differences from men; others de-emphasized gender differences. Once the necessary changes were made, it is clear that employers planned to treat men and women equally with respect to the physical environment.

Techniques to integrate women quickly into the workforce began with pre-employment physical examinations that screened for contagious disease, a variety of physical defects, and chronic diseases like emphysema or asthma. Many workers were opposed to these exams, believing that their findings could be unfairly used. The Oregon State Board of Health even viewed male and female worker resistance as an obstacle to coordinated planning for wartime health and safety.[9]

But some women workers wanted more complete physical examinations to prove their strength and ability. A group of welders in Oregon believed that if physicians properly tested all employees before starting work, the ones with "weak lungs" would be weeded out and not go on to develop respiratory diseases that could be unfairly blamed on welding. More than one personnel director agreed with the War Manpower Commission that renewed attention to the pre-employment exam, which emphasized a woman's physical condition rather than her age, and focused on matching her to the physical requirement of the jobs, would result in a "steadier employee." This use of the exam would undoubtedly influence standards for selecting men as well.[10]

Once hired, women resembled other new employees. Insurance executives predicted that accident rates would be higher because these women lacked experience—not because they were women. The training of women workers, however, often followed traditional gender assumptions by suggesting that women's concern with femininity risked the safety of male workers. Employers wanted "gals" to look like "guys."[11] Women received training that firmly reminded them to hide their bodies. Accompanying new female hires on a plant tour, a manager at a West Coast aircraft company reportedly pointed out a man working on a drill press who had lost three fingers when he became distracted by one woman's inappropriately feminine work costume. Whether or not this story is true, the fact is that many managers remained unconvinced that men and women could safely work in the same space unless the "defeminization" of women workers was as complete as possible. Other employers had a more upbeat view, believing that women not only responded well to safety regulations but that their "natural cautiousness" had a positive influence on their male co-workers.[12] Against the onslaught of new workers, veteran male workers undoubtedly increased their own attention to safety, careful to be on guard against the lapses in judgement and clumsiness that often accompanied inexperience.

Employers hoped that proper safety equipment and clothing would adequately protect women, although, again, assumptions about women's concern with fashion created a variety of strategies to ensure compliance. While many supervisors noted that women followed health and safety regulations more scrupulously than men, this happened in spite of women's perceived concerns about personal appearance, which should have made them reluctant to wear goggles or caps that hid their hair.[13]

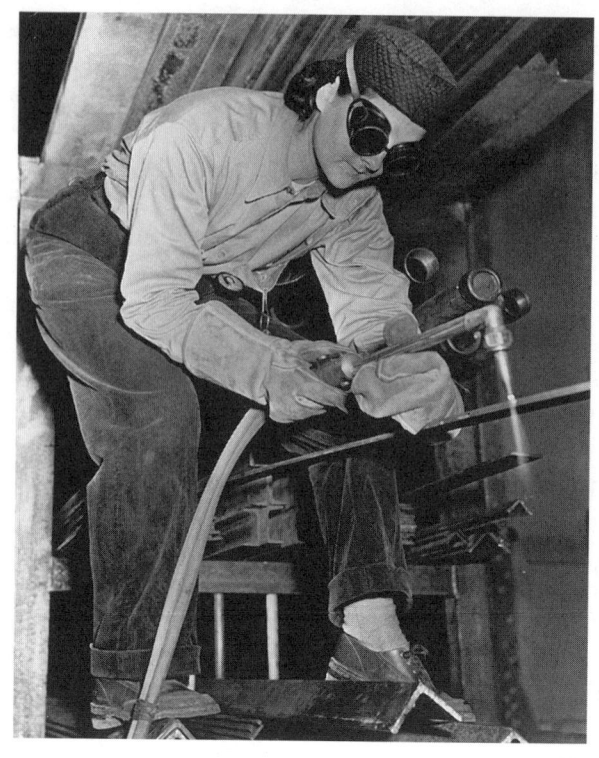

A welder in the South Carolina Navy Yard during World War II.

The National Safety Council used fear to send a message about the dangers of "loose flowing hair" in the workplace: "accidents of this kind always leave an unsightly scar." The secretary of labor, Frances Perkins, also warned women to wear head protection, but claimed she was more concerned about reports of accidents caused by women wearing high-heeled shoes. "The accidents to women fall largely into the 'slip, fall, and stumble' category," Perkins told a New York Women's Trade Union League conference. Such accidents could be prevented by wearing low-heeled shoes.[14]

Some employers resorted to embarrassment to enforce proper behavior. The medical director of a cigar factory more accustomed to women workers offered this advice: when a woman worker who was walking downstairs lost both heels of her shoes and broke her coccyx, "Those shoes were paraded in a truck through the plant, together with a pair of work shoes."[15]

Women workers defied these stereotypes. Juanita Loveless, a welder at Vega Aircraft in California, recalled that many of her female co-workers had no problem cutting their hair short: "[Otherwise], your hair would slip down and you'd try to get it up, and your hands were filthy with chemicals and little bits of metal. It was like rubbing salt into a wound." Similar attitudes about shoes could be found among women workers at the Todd Shipyards. The personnel director, Elinore Herrick, admitted that when she and her staff researched the "best" safety shoes for women, fashion had been an important consideration. But when the shoes arrived, the women refused to wear them because the soles were too thin and the shoes afforded no protection to the ankles. They wanted equal treatment—and equal protection. They rejected the shoes because they had no steel toe or shank, declaring, "We want steel toes like the men." Herrick sent the shoes back, but she still worried that the smallest men's shoes would "ruin the women's feet, with their higher arches and their long use of relatively high heels." As it happened, only an extra pair of socks was needed to provide an adequate fit for those "unshapely, hulking men's shoes." Other workers chose a middle route, refusing to accept completely male-defined workplace standards. Recognizing real hazards on the job, some kept their hair out of the way with colorful scarves and bandeaux when doing so did not compromise other safety requirements.[16]

When not judging women on their fashion sense, employers recognized physical differences between men and women and adjusted work processes and machinery at their plants in order to accommodate women's differences in height, weight, and upper body strength relative to men's. The Frankford Arsenal in Philadelphia subdivided its work making fuses, which allowed the Army to make the best use of women's smaller fingers. Women themselves contributed to the efforts to change the work, as Mabel Maddox at Curtiss-Wright in Ohio demonstrated. Maddox invented a rotating jig to hold and move one type of gas tank while welding it. A manager at Marinship Company in California praised a man who designed a narrow-handled scraper blade handle that better fit the hands of women, who were experiencing hand cramps from using traditional paint scrapers.[17]

Employers perceived the biggest problem to be the reduction of heavy lifting in many industrial jobs, the hazards of which had long been a source of concern to labor reformers. During the war, one industrial nurse noted that menstrual periods lasted longer among women who did heavier work. In addition to reproductive abnormalities, lifting risked harm to muscles and ligaments in bodies not accustomed to hefting heavy weights and also led to dropping hazards, endangering bones as well as nearby workers. Well before the war, many states had enacted maximum weight laws. In some states women were prohibited from lifting more than twenty-five pounds, in others fifteen pounds, and in still others fifty pounds. Companies with plants in more than one state had found such laws inefficient, and while some of them challenged the laws on a state-by-state basis, others chose to adjust the workplace in an effort to regularize production, even though the war emergency had allowed the rescinding of some of these weight limits. Companies developed overhead lifting devices and other mechanical moving equipment, as well as staging instead of ladders. Herrick at the Todd Shipyards believed that in the long run re-engineering would also benefit men: it let "brains supplant brawn."[18]

As production picked up, companies began to rely more on each worker's individual characteristics and suitability for particular jobs and put less credence in gender stereotypes. They recognized what many workers—male and female—already knew: some women were stronger and more capable than some men, and vice versa. Such insights revealed flaws in protective labor laws, especially with respect to weight lifting. One woman at the Monarch Machine Tool Company in Ohio resisted efforts to move her off an assembly job simply because it required her to lift pieces that weighed close to the twenty-five-pound limit specified by the state. To some women these laws defied logic. Mothers accustomed to lifting and carrying children were presumably capable of transferring that skill to the workplace.[19]

Overall, employers temporarily adapted the workplace to accommodate women workers. Many of the adaptations involved re-engineering machinery and industrial processes. Other changes did not so much adapt as extend common personnel practices. Retooling and examinations de-emphasized women's physical deviation from men's abilities and supported employers' desires to stress individual responsibility for health and safety. Employers clearly expected that women would perform as adequately as men. Drawing on women's own attitudes toward equality, managers said they wanted women who were "loath to complain, to act the cry baby, or to do anything that would bring discredit to their sex." For their part, many women expected neither favors nor discrimination from employers and male co-workers because of their sex. The historian Sherna Berger Gluck has argued that the wartime work experiences allowed women to "hold their own with men."[20]

Holding their own also meant taking an equal risk of exposure to hazardous materials. Harder to regulate and control than machinery, these dangers were sometimes less easily recognized, producing delayed symptoms. Efforts to reduce exposure to hazardous materials had typically centered on mechanical ventilation and personal protective equipment. Women, like their male counterparts, used materials that were known to cause both acute and chronic respiratory problems or were suspected to be carcinogenic. At a Bath Iron Works prefabricating plant in Brunswick, Maine, for example, women used asbestos to wrap pipes. They also sewed tea cozy–like asbestos pads to fit over valves.[21]

Fumes from welding in shipyards and aircraft plants occurred as a result of the interaction of a variety of metals. Some women believed themselves to be more subject to such fumes than men, not because of any inherent female weakness but because of where they worked on the ship. "The air got thicker and thicker," recalled one welder, "and of course up near the ceiling where I worked, it was the worst." The men did not notice it, she said, because "they didn't work up near the ceiling." Women welders demanded proper protection from hazardous fumes. In a voice that reflected the employer rhetoric of personal responsibility, Augusta Clawson, an Oregon shipyard welder, demanded air pipes when welding in a poorly ventilated space, declaring it to be "our own fault when we get 'welder's wheeze.'"[22]

The Women's Bureau opposed the employer strategy of allowing women to take equal risks and responsibilities for protecting their health. It trusted neither women nor employers and instead tried to mandate additional protection beyond state legislation. But although the bureau attempted to prohibit women from working with a wide variety of substances, including mercury, arsenic, and silica, Alice Hamilton urged the bureau's director, Mary Anderson, not to because those materials were "no more harmful for women than for men."[23] Few were willing to exempt women from handling hazardous materials if doing so would hinder the war effort.

Surprisingly, employers and the medical community somewhat successfully applied this strategy of equal risk even when dealing with pregnancy and reproduction. In contrast to the conventional wisdom of the period, many supported the assertions of one employment manual that "many women have proved to be much more valuable employees before or after the birth of the child if they are permitted to work for a reasonable length of time." Employers did not automatically reject or fire pregnant women, although disagreement surfaced around this issue. Many personnel managers urged the transfer of pregnant women to less hazardous work if necessary, but some did not agree. Virginia Lemire at the Kaiser Company in Portland, Oregon, believed that transferring pregnant women to more suitable jobs in the yard imposed undue interference on production. She urged pregnant women to quit or take leaves of absence. Her comments indicate more concern about the disruption of production than about potential health risks to women.[24]

Women's Bureau researchers tried to steer employers away from placing pregnant women in certain jobs, especially those that required heavy lifting. They argued that pregnancy caused a "noticeable compression on the heart." At this point the surgeon general, O. F. Hedley, entered the debate, disagreeing and explaining that while pregnancy did increase the work of the heart and displaced it upward and laterally, it did not actually compress it. In fact, he reported, most obstetricians believed that a "moderate degree of physical exercise" by pregnant women, including a certain amount of weight lifting, produced less painful labor and delivery. Within reasonable limits, he argued, weight lifting was not injurious.[25]

Interestingly, the bureau and the surgeon general appeared to switch sides over the importance of pelvic exams in employment and placement exams. Hedley argued that a woman's gynecological history should be a significant hiring factor, especially when she would be expected to perform heavy lifting, but he qualified his concerns. "Where there is a past history of pregnancy or tumors," said Hedley, employers should establish a firm policy regarding "the interval between pregnancy and employment involving heavy lifting." In this, Hedley was firmly in the company of many industrial physicians, who spent a lot of time persuading women of the value of such exams. Physicians, however, denied having any discriminatory motives. At United Aircraft, one claimed that he treated a woman with "pelvic pathology" the same as he treated a man with a hernia.[26]

The Women's Bureau approached equality a little differently. It supported pre-employment exams but, walking a fine line between discrimination and protection, tried to discourage overemphasis on pelvic exams because it believed that they might highlight female differences. It is not entirely clear why Hedley was more concerned with postpartum women than pregnant women, but the Women's Bureau's behavior is more easily explained. Dogged by the National Woman's Party for its opposition to the ERA and support for protective legislation, the bureau trod carefully when it came to employment policies that might be construed as limiting women's employment opportunities. As a result, pregnancy policies across the country varied—as did the bureau's responses to them—but all of them indicated some loosening of previous restrictions.

Pregnant or not, women of childbearing age also risked reproductive harm from a variety of chemicals in the wartime workplace. Lead was a well-known hazard. Most of the lead poisoning in shipyards resulted from contact with lead paint, made by adding benzene in kegs to red lead powder. At Marinship in California, women painted joints, valves, and ventilators, as well as compartments and bottoms, with lead paint. Women used solid lead for soldering and molten lead for pouring molds and making alloys, all activities that released lead fumes. Chippers and caulkers used red lead packing between plates. As early as 1918, Hamilton had recommended that because of lead's reproductive dangers, some women should be prohibited from working in certain industrial processes. Employers downplayed this prescription during World War II in favor of urging workers to take greater personal responsibility for their health.[27]

Shipyards encouraged the use of respirators for women working on galvanized metal or on surfaces painted with red lead, just as they had long done for

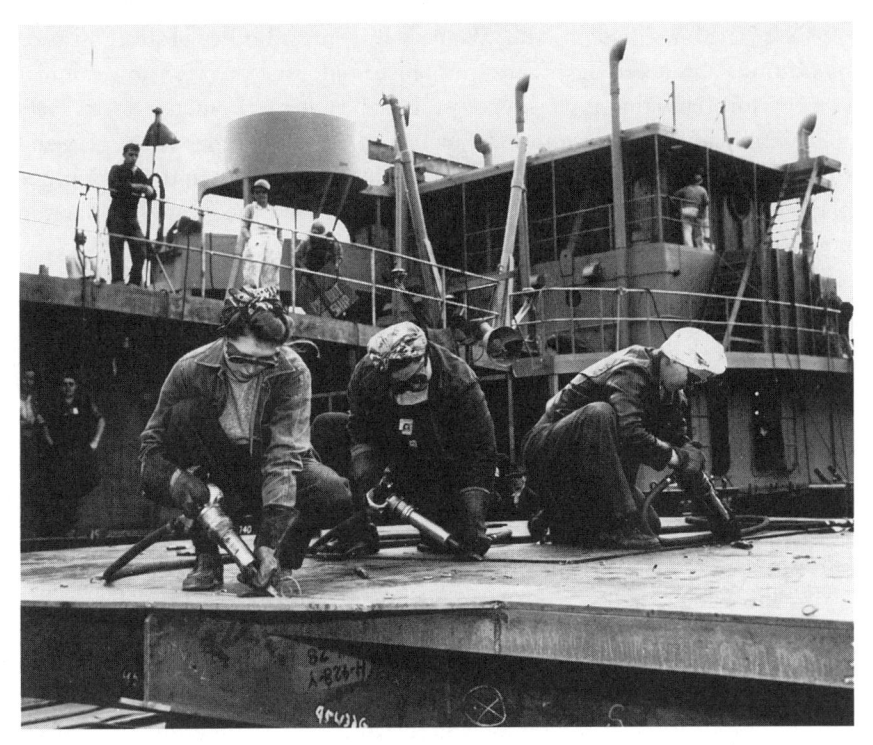

Chippers removing red lead paint at Marinship, Sausalito, California, in 1942.

male workers. Workers were also urged to keep their hands clean and not to eat lunch in the workroom. Frequent blood counts provided an indication of the lead in each worker's system and, at the first sign of lead poisoning, most plant physicians suggested transferring affected workers.[28]

Hamilton had studied lead poisoning for more than thirty years and took its effects on women's reproductive abilities seriously, but she also carefully and deliberately did not overstate reproductive dangers to women in industry. When Women's Bureau officials tried to publish a list of hazards from which women should be specifically excluded, she persuaded them to focus only on the reproductive dangers, which she believed were limited to lead and benzene. Hamilton and others had written widely on women's increased susceptibility to lead and benzene poisoning, in addition to the reproductive hazards they posed, but in a speech shortly after the war ended, she admitted that "careful observation of large groups in the poisonous trades" indicated otherwise. Age, for example, had seemed to be more of a factor in benzene poisoning, with young (menstruating) women more susceptible than young men, although even this assertion was under scrutiny.[29]

Despite efforts made by the Women's Bureau and other protectionists to be cautious about certain hazards, employers adopted their by now familiar strategy for maintaining workplace health and safety. Women workers were told about industrial poisons and then urged to wear proper safety gear and to maintain proper personal hygiene, keeping hair, hands, and clothing free of chemicals and hazardous substances. This allowed for greater production potential.

Employers and medical professionals also responded to feminist notions of equality. After the temporary lifting of state protective laws, the National Association of Manufacturers wondered if "it might be wise to repeal protective legislation entirely, trusting the women to make their own rules as they go along, just as men do." The National Woman's Party agreed. It believed that the wartime employment of women would prove women capable of performing a wide variety of jobs without harm to themselves or their families. Both groups had supported the ERA since its first introduction in 1923. In pursuit of their goals, the National Woman's Party had placed continual pressure on the protectionist Women's Bureau for twenty years.[30]

Public health officials, obstetricians and gynecologists, and industrial physicians likewise moved between reducing differential treatment of male and female workers and recognizing differences. At a 1943 medical symposium on the "Health of Women Industry," Milton Kronenberg of the Illinois Department of Public Hygiene said he believed that certain jobs and working conditions were not suited to women largely due to "limitations of physique, biologic differences, and experience." But he emphasized that the workplace environment should be made "equally safe for men and for women. . . . Poor working conditions have no sex differential."[31]

Some conditions did have a sex differential. Menstrual cramps exasperated industrial physicians. "Epidemic dysmenorrhea" resulted in a great deal of lost time and interruption of production, according to Max Burnell of General Motors. He and other physicians recommended that workers not be sent home (as they had apparently successfully requested while in school) but instead be provided with exercises and information on proper diet and posture. One physician claimed to reduce absences due to dysmenorrhea by "checking up on repeaters." A consultant for the industry's Industrial Hygiene Foundation wondered if "a certain number of cases of dysmenorrhea may be an excuse . . . for absence."[32]

Paying attention to physical and sex differences resulted in limited accommodations by employers. But the reality of women's social differences elicited a different response, at least initially. At the same symposium that Kronenberg attended, a New York physician expressed amazement at what women had done but argued that "more attention must be paid to a woman's outside activities and responsibilities than has ever been paid to a man's. . . . These mothers and wives often work as many hours at home as at the plant." This was not news to women wage-earners. A woman who worked nights at northern New Jersey's Picatinny Arsenal complained that men on her shift could go to bed when they finished work, while women had "home and family to attend to." She wondered if women were indeed the "weaker sex."[33]

Women workers demanded that employers recognize those socially determined domestic roles, and they gave voice to their demands by calling in sick. Absenteeism in war-related industries was higher among women than among men. At Marinship women composed 20 percent of the workforce but accounted for 37 percent of the absenteeism in 1943. At least one other California shipbuilding employer wondered if shipyard jobs were "too hard for women." Employers who read Women's Bureau reports might have found some support for this position. Despite efforts to increase employment of women in many war-related industries, bureau investigators used scientific evidence to argue that women tended to "tire more quickly," that constant standing was "more difficult and harmful" for women, and indeed, that the confusion and din of the shipyards tired women out. So did climbing and crouching in and around the ships.[34]

The inability of employers to understand the reasons behind high absenteeism can also be seen in their determined efforts to ignore women's off-the-clock lives as much as possible. Several employment manuals told new hires that "home troubles must be left at home," but many working women ignored that advice. They demanded that employers consider other conditions that affected on-the-job performance, notably fatigue. Remember Alma, whose household responsibilities interrupted her sleep on a regular basis? She showed up for work an hour before her shift began because, she said, her husband would not go to bed while she was at home, and she felt he needed his sleep.[35]

Attempts to quantify fatigue had attracted the attention of social reformers years before World War II. While the research had failed to identify fatigue definitively as a medical fact, empirical evidence from a variety of sources indicated that health and work performance suffered when people were tired. Lower resistance increased likelihood of disease. Heavier breathing led to more toxic exposure. Poor blood circulation led to mistakes. Ignored nutritional demands slowed mental and physical reaction times. It was by no means a stretch for contemporary observers to understand that women's double duty created the conditions for absenteeism. As one employment counselor mused, "The wonder is that the rate is not much higher, when you consider that they are working perhaps sixteen hours a day in the yard and at home."[36]

Despite a long tradition of various forms of industrial welfarism, employers had little experience with these types of non-occupational factors directly affecting workplace health. Here determined efforts by managers to treat women and men equally did not entirely work. Faced with high absenteeism, how did employers respond? Many felt they could not afford to let women's maternal duties interfere with production and hired "woman counselors" who were expected to smooth the adjustment from housewife to factory worker, interpret company rules and regulations, help with housing and child care, establish recreational activities, act as a troubleshooter and sympathetic listener, and advise on diet and health. The successful counselor, usually not a supervisor but a member of the personnel department, was hired to help the employer maintain high production through low turnover and low absenteeism.[37]

The woman counselor was not a medical professional, because most employers did not see the problems of female absenteeism as exclusively or even primarily medical. Accustomed to understanding medicine as a profession of many specialties, employers looked at health more in terms of disease, that is, specific pathogens that manifested certain symptoms and could be treated by the application of certain therapies. Employers preferred to consider absenteeism a personnel rather than a medical problem.[38]

Nevertheless, several counselors identified fatigue as the major cause of health factors resulting in female absenteeism. Citing the double duty of many married women like Alma, several woman counselors believed that "women workers are likely to succumb to fatigue if they have . . . household chores to perform in addition to the regular hours of work." Among East Coast shipyard workers, one survey attributed over 75 percent of female absences to "illness and fatigue" and "home conditions." Kaiser, which operated shipyards on the West Coast, surveyed four hundred of its "worst absentees" among women workers and described nearly half as "physically exhausted and in desperate need of medical attention." Susan Laughlin, a counselor at Lockheed in California, investigated absences that turned out to be nutritionally related: "You'd find women cooking for their children and not wanting to eat."[39]

Solutions varied. A Marinship counselor, Marcia Patterson, recommended action that went well beyond changing the workplace: provide child care and persuade stores and dentists to stay open late. In many cases counselors acted as advocates for women workers as they dealt with school boards and other institutions. Still others made referrals for abortions, still illegal in the 1940s.[40]

Perhaps recognizing the limits of their influence, many counselors turned to solutions that more closely reflected employer attempts to redirect responsibility for fatigue-induced illness. Some blamed the tired worker for having too many dates or attending too many parties and made unfavorable comparisons to productive and hardworking German and Japanese women. Others encouraged women to adopt sound management strategies at home: better organization and careful planning of household duties through "wiser use of time," delegating authority, and seeking "expert advice" on housework. Failing that, this group of personnel counselors urged the hiring of maids, which may have been helpful to some of the growing number of middle-class women workers but did little to alleviate the household duties of millions of working-class white and African-American women who could not afford to hire help. Indeed, many of these war workers had left domestic employment themselves in order to seek better, more lucrative work.[41]

Virginia Lemire of Kaiser was completely disgusted after reviewing the "worst absentees" among women workers at Kaiser's Swan Island yard in Oregon. Good use of pre-employment examinations and interviews, she argued, would have prevented the hiring of workers with big families. The company should be "eliminating these people from working," Lemire wrote, because those were the women absent most often. She cited women with three or four children who took time off because of a variety of common but serious illnesses that affected their children.[42]

Counselors, regardless of their opinions about women's fatigue, made two important contributions to the workplace with respect to occupational health. They recognized that some women did carry different burdens from men's. By emphasizing personal responsibility, however, counselors ultimately buttressed employer efforts first to recognize and then to reduce the significance of wage-earning women's social duties.

Nevertheless, it is important to see that working women related to their environment differently from the way men did. In so doing, women were attempting to redefine workplace health, even if few recognized it at the time. Women in war-related industries did not ask for a different work environment; instead they wanted help in handling their nonwork environment. This meant that wartime workers and employers alike felt the impact of ideas about equality and difference in the workplace. Women workers felt the often divergent and contradictory outcomes in their own lives and health. Being treated no differently from male workers furthered an argument in favor of gender equality but ignored the variety of women's social roles. Employers recognized the economic advantages of promoting equality when it came to health measures. The great irony of women's workplace experiences during World War II, at least when viewed from the perspective of occupational safety and health, is that women themselves undermined much of the basis for protective laws but developed few organized strategies to force employers to continue to account for socially prescribed differences between men and women.[43]

Women began to lose defense-related jobs even before the war ended, but the significance of their experiences reveals the advantages and the limits of equality in changing women's position in the workforce and in redefining workplace health. Both of these issues speak to contemporary health debates. By the end of the war the legitimacy of protective labor laws had been severely tested, but many of the strongest proponents of these laws had always viewed special legislation as a means to an end. When women and men were provided the same tools, instructions, and personal protective equipment, it became clear that differences between individual men and women were more real than those between men and women as groups, and once physical characteristics rather than gender determined job suitability, protective labor laws seemed less defensible.

Employers liked the idea of equality because it gave them more choices in hiring. It also reduced the need to adjust the workplace environment to fit the worker, women having proved themselves as capable as men without protective labor laws. While wartime circumstances did compel some employers to re-engineer the workplace in order to rely less on individual strength alone, for the most part, having women in the workplace resulted in few long-term health and safety changes. Integration largely meant acceptance of existing standards. The burden for maintaining health could be shifted too easily to the worker, with the employer absolved of maintaining adequate working conditions. And workers' freedoms could be restricted because chronic illnesses or defects would prevent them from being hired.

5
Alice Hamilton and the Equal Rights Amendment

In the years after World War II, attitudes about the Equal Rights Amendment shifted. Alice Hamilton dropped her opposition to the ERA in 1952, to the delight of the National Woman's Party and the distress of the National Consumers' League. She said she now believed that the health of American working women was too much in the public eye to be ignored, which is what many opponents of the ERA originally feared would occur if the amendment became law. Hamilton had seen "so great a change in the position of women workers in the last 15 years or so" that she thought an ERA would merely confirm an equality between men and women that had "already been largely achieved."[1]

While some of these changes can be attributed to workplace modifications brought about by World War II, Hamilton took a longer view. She spoke as a social reformer, a woman who had spent more than thirty years of her life as a member of the National Consumers' League—four of them as its president, and several more as vice president. Like many National Consumers' League members, Hamilton had opposed a constitutional amendment that would provide "equal rights" for women, something many agreed had not been achieved with female suffrage, and she had disagreed with the prime movers of the amendment, the National Woman's Party, every time it was introduced in the United States Congress, beginning in 1923. Like many Progressive Era activists, she had believed that industrial conditions in the early years of the twentieth century were bad for workers' health, and especially bad for the masses of women relegated to low-paying, unskilled jobs. Hamilton had seen how low wages and lack of skills both limited working women's opportunities and led to their overwork. She had supported legislation to prevent employers from exploiting women's relative political and economic weaknesses in the paid workforce and to provide time for working women to perform household and child-rearing responsibilities.

Hamilton was also a physician, an industrial toxicologist who had investigated workplace hazards for more than forty years. Her medical training led her to seek out physiological explanations for such diseases as benzene poisoning. In the 1920s, for instance, she had refused to take a position on the regulation of

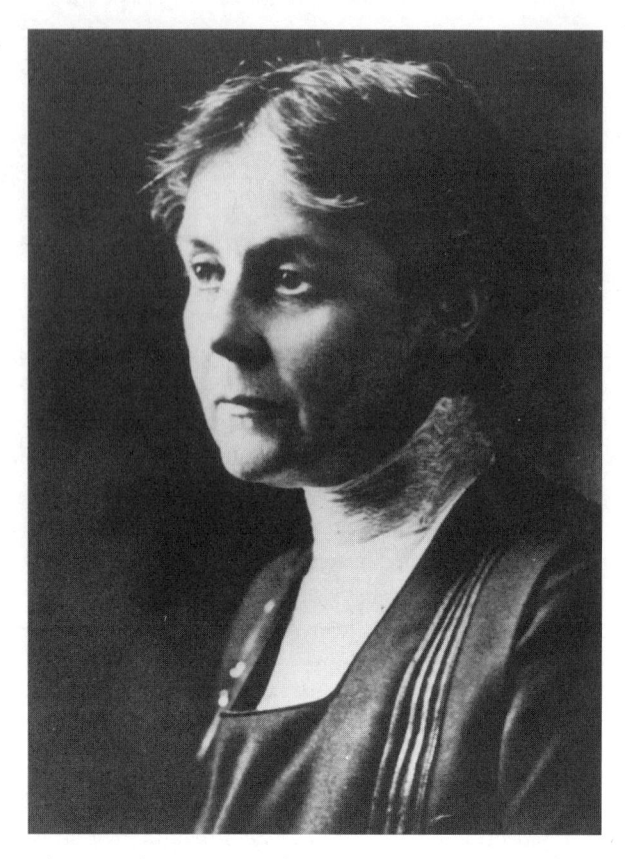

Alice Hamilton, M.D., industrial toxicologist and professor of public health at Harvard University. 1919 photo taken from a print at Francis A. Countway Library of Medicine, Boston, Massachusetts.

benzene in the workplace until she could identify the blood changes that it caused and explain its differential effects on men, women, and young girls.[2] Hamilton's social awareness of the relationship between health and environment and her professional understanding of modern science gave her a unique perspective on the conditions of women in industry.

What changed her mind? Why did this protectionist former president of the National Consumers' League drop her opposition to the ERA? Hamilton had supported two different kinds of protective legislation—each the result of her particular experiences—and distinguished between them. As a physician trained in modern scientific theory and practice, Hamilton believed that society had an interest in protecting women from those hazards "that were more injurious to women than to men," or those that affected women's ability to bear healthy children. She most frequently cited lead. In such cases she based the exclusion of women from certain jobs on a biological understanding of differences between men and women, suggesting narrower parameters of protection than those that simply shortened the number of hours women could work.[3]

But Hamilton had rooted her support for limiting hours in her experiences as an investigator and social reformer, where she had witnessed firsthand the deleterious effects of women's double duty. Aware that double duty constituted an integral part of most working women's lives, Hamilton believed that protective labor laws benefited not only working women but also a society that still viewed a woman's primary role as that of homemaker. Practicality also guided her; results from state factory investigations had persuaded her of the need to improve conditions for all workers, but if protecting no workers was the only alternative, she recognized the benefits of protecting women workers at least. During the first third of the century, few feminists on either side of the protective labor legislation issue made the complex distinctions that Hamilton recognized.

Eventually, however, Hamilton's perception of the need for hours laws changed, leaving only her concern for the biological effects of individual hazards. To look at this intellectual shift is to understand the impact of the ERA on women's workplace health in the twentieth century, especially from the 1920s through World War II. Ultimately the pro-ERA arguments reduced the legitimacy of rationales that had been used to protect all women in favor of looking at individual rather than group characteristics for employment suitability. While this provided more job opportunities to women, especially in nontraditional, higher-paying jobs, it also opened a door for new policies of exclusion based on women's reproductive capacity, whose results created an array of new and potentially divisive challenges for feminists and women workers in the 1960s and 1970s.

Pro- and anti-ERA feminists agreed on some basic biological issues, but their differences parallel divergent ideas about medicine, the role of public health in society, and the relative importance of individual over categorical distinctions. The intersection of gender with medicine, with World War II, and with capitalism created more complex and diverse notions of motherhood, providing the basis for the change in Hamilton's thinking. Her views became a bridge for an eventual convergence of opinion about the ERA in the 1960s. Understanding the feminist roots of protective labor legislation illuminates the variety of feminisms that continued to influence workplace health policies.

Feminists who had unified around female suffrage disagreed sharply over the benefits that an ERA would bring to U.S. women. The proposed ERA mandated gender equality under the law, while gender-based state protective laws treated women workers differently from their male counterparts. Two realities of working women's experiences had convinced some feminists of the need for protective laws: (1) the wage work of many women, unlike some men, often occurred under unorganized, low-paying, and dirty conditions; and (2) married working women were responsible for the various household tasks in their families, also unlike many similarly situated men. Protective laws were presumed to have achieved the same rights for women that male workers had won through unionizing. They prevented a woman's overwork to the detriment of family and society.[4]

Activists on both sides believed that the passage of an ERA would eliminate protective laws. Feminist supporters of the ERA believed that such laws legitimated gender inequality in the workplace. Women would never be considered equal to men, they argued, as long as state labor laws decreed women incapable of making their own decisions about employment.[5]

Both sides claimed that concerns about women's health informed their positions, but ERA supporters had challenged protectionists to demonstrate that protective labor legislation, which arguably targeted only a small segment of society—namely, married women—improved the health and welfare of all women. Speaking before a 1926 luncheon to introduce the Women's Bureau of the National Association of Manufacturers, Ada R. Wolff had quoted vital statistics from states with restrictive laws and those without, and asked, "Does any of you really believe that the women of Illinois, Florida, and North Carolina are less healthy than those of Massachusetts, Pennsylvania and New Jersey?" Weight-lifting restrictions for women seemed equally unscientific and not properly based on notions of women's health, according to Dr. R. A. Spaeth of Johns Hopkins University. Empirical evidence during World War I had made it clear to Spaeth that despite a variety of weight restrictions in many states (which in itself suggested a lack of scientific standards unless one assumed that, to appropriate Wolff's analogy, women were weaker in certain states), women could successfully lift well over those limits. He had argued that when scientific studies established employment requirements for all jobs, men's and women's health would be equally ensured against industrial hazards.[6]

ERA supporters believed that women's abilities to make choices based on their own social, economic, and personal needs would be enhanced by the amendment's passage. In 1924 Bryn Mawr College's president, M. Carey Thomas, had couched her support in the context of liberal, laissez-faire individualism: "How much better by one blow to do away with discriminating against women in work, salaries, promotion and opportunities to compete with men in a fair field with no favour on either side!"[7]

Protectionists not surprisingly pointed out the material conditions of working women's home and factory lives. They urged the public to recognize the special health needs of women who worked in dirty, dusty conditions and who found the monotonous work fatiguing. All of this also hindered women's ability to do housework and take care of children. Women in the textile mills of New Jersey experienced deafening noise, excessive heat and humidity, long hours of standing, and high-speed machinery during the night shift. As one mill worker had admitted to Agnes deLima of the National Consumers' League: "Plenty womans get sick, die maybe, so much work." Protectionists distrusted capitalist employers or employer associations like the Industrial Council of Passaic (New Jersey) Wool Manufacturers, who they believed would exploit women if they could. Protectionists believed that protective laws would help women maintain sufficient health to do both jobs. The impetus for better health, they argued, should come from the state, not from women's individual efforts.[8]

Professional women, however, would benefit from an ERA. Largely unaffected by protective laws, these women stood to gain from the increased educational and employment opportunities that would presumably accrue to them after an ERA was enacted. Protectionists, many of them professional women themselves, had nevertheless tried to encourage their sisters to ignore these class divisions in favor of gender solidarity. This strategy had worked in a few cases, but when it failed, protectionists branded all ERA supporters as elite professional women blind to the real needs of working-class women. In the early postsuffrage years, for instance, medical women had responded favorably to the arguments of their protectionist colleague Hamilton. Hoping she could appeal to the humanitarian side of women physicians, Hamilton had decided to confront this group's class concerns head-on. At the 1924 annual meeting of the Medical Women's National Association, she had urged the board of directors to ignore "whatever privileges [the ERA] might bring to the better class of women," and to "think of the great body of inarticulate, helpless working women." Hamilton supported a motion that the Medical Women's National Association join the Women's Joint Congressional Committee, which lobbied on behalf of women's issues, and support its legislative agenda, including opposition to the ERA.[9]

Hamilton's impassioned appeal to the entire organization prompted its president, Dr. Esther Lovejoy, to call immediately for a resolution opposing the ERA. This resolution passed almost unanimously. The Medical Women's National Association's public opposition to the ERA lasted only about four years, however, which is not surprising, given the organization's professional membership. Moreover, women doctors became aware of a previously unrecognized indirect economic link that would cause them to rethink their position. In the 1930s the editor of *The Medical Women's Journal* warned female physicians that the passage of hours and minimum wage legislation for industrial women might, by reducing these women's overall income, also materially reduce the income that women doctors would receive from working-class patients and their families. The Medical Women's National Association's emergence (under its new name, the American Medical Women's Association) as a strong supporter of the ERA during World War II was what had prompted the National Consumers' League to recruit Hamilton to write an anti-ERA article. Ironically, this article led to her reversal of opinion about the amendment.[10]

While equal rights feminists appeared willing to adopt some of the language of protectionist feminists, judgments about who was protected by labor laws and from which workplace hazards women needed protection had differed markedly. Protectionists believed that state labor laws kept married women safe for motherhood by protecting women from overwork and the other excesses of industrial capitalism. To protectionists, safety involved prevention of fatigue from overlong hours, which would enable women to bear healthy children and to rear them in a wholesome household and a hygienic community. Such laws also kept single women "safe" until marriage and motherhood. In 1912 the National Consumers' League researcher Josephine Goldmark had argued that "the strain of continuous standing and overwork during girlhood, such as many young women endure in stores as well as factories [was] responsible for unmistakable pelvic and uterine disease and sometimes sterility after marriage." To Mary van Kleeck fourteen years later, protection meant freedom. Since women had different social experiences from men's, as well as less power to control their environment, they had less freedom. Van Kleeck believed that the community should act to control these conditions, allowing individuals to experience "more, not less, freedom" to be women.[11]

Pro-ERA forces, however, had countered that protectionists promoted discriminatory legislation, that protective laws in fact protected men's jobs from women who wanted better jobs, such as making metal molds in foundries. They could point to the New York State Factory Investigating Commission's conclusion in 1912 that conditions in core-making rooms posed hazards for both men and women. The commission had expressed regret that women had ever been allowed to do this work, and the commissioners advocated the prohibition of women from this work for the benefit of the race. This fell in line with the goal of the all-male molders' union.[12]

Furthermore, equal rights feminists believed that protective laws showed obvious selectivity and were often enforced according to community needs. A British physician recounted a conversation with an American reformer at the 1926 Women's Industrial Conference sponsored by the Women's Bureau. The American had supported night work restrictions for women. "'Then we will have no night nurses?' [asked the British woman.] 'Oh, yes,' replied the reformer. 'Of course, we must have night nurses.'" Even Hamilton had remarked how agricultural and domestic workers, whose tasks were at least as strenuous as, if not more strenuous than, several manufacturing jobs, often found themselves excluded from protective labor laws.[13]

Although feminists in the 1920s and beyond disagreed over how best to promote working women's health, modern scientific medicine provided the intellectual underpinnings for both sides. On the one hand, the new medical emphasis on individual responsibility, as set in place by employers and public health officials beginning in the 1920s, strengthened the position of equal rights feminists, who believed that individual characteristics rather than gender notions would advance women's socioeconomic position. On the other hand, feminists who believed that protective legislation improved women's lives used physiological evidence supplied by industrial physicians on women's strength, resistance to disease and, most important, reproductive function, to argue that a number of industrial conditions uniquely threatened women.

Where industrial poisons were concerned, a close examination of the arguments about physiology demonstrates similar concerns among advocates on both sides of the ERA. Frances Perkins, who had been a factory inspector, was forthright for a protectionist in 1926:

> It is my opinion that very few of the strictly prohibitory laws are justified by facts. . . . A few relate to occupations believed to be hazardous to health. . . . The cure for this kind of industrial risk is better sanitary measures, not prohibition. In cases where a health hazard affects women peculiarly—and such [sic] exists in connection with some chemicals—prohibition is justified.[14]

Elizabeth Faulkner Baker, Perkins's opponent in this debate, was equally specific, acknowledging that some prohibitory laws had been justified for health reasons. But she argued that industrial engineering had sufficiently changed working conditions to allow women to be hired for these jobs.[15]

This common understanding of industrial hazards underscores how closely many of these feminists resembled one another, especially given the fact that many National Woman's Party members, including its president, Alice Paul, had once supported protective legislation. Moreover, although few feminists admitted it, agreeing to acknowledge sexual distinctions regarding industrial poisons and, more important, agreeing to consider pregnancy and maternity legislation separately, also suggests a common understanding of motherhood. Wendy Sarvasy has argued that in the 1920s both groups of feminists believed that upholding motherhood was important in achieving their common goal of what she has called a "feminist welfare state." While anti-ERA forces had advocated mothers' pensions as an entering wedge for universal entitlements for married women, for example, ERA supporters had envisioned such pensions in the context of similar programs for soldiers.[16]

Feminists in the 1920s had largely ignored these points because, in fact, biological realities complicated the arguments both for and against protection. Even when people did not know the precise way in which lead affected women's reproductive functions, for instance, they knew that biological changes occurred from exposure to lead, the effects of which were most visible in the sex that carried the child in utero. Biological and physiological differences between men and women were hard to ignore. But pro-ERA feminists only reluctantly mentioned biological differences. They feared acknowledging them lent credence to the anti-ERA view that because women were different, that they needed special consideration, that they were somehow unequal.

Yet the emphasis on biology ultimately strengthened pro-ERA arguments that women need not be subject to broad-based laws that governed all industrial conditions. Employment standards could instead compel employers to consider differences in work requirements and in individual strengths or capabilities. Such policies, like protective labor laws, might treat women as a group, but they could focus more on the individual processes within industry rather than on social distinctions between men and women. Hamilton had taken this position in a very early example of such specific attention to workplace hazards, stating in 1917 that, "so long as the danger is one which a man faces equally, I think there is no reason why a woman should not face it also."[17] For a protectionist, her assessment seems remarkably individualist, and she encouraged even more attention to specific job characteristics and job processes during and after World War II.

For the anti-ERA feminists, biological differences constituted a solid basis for protective legislation. Focusing on differences bolstered the "women are different" argument. One could easily conduct studies "proving" the relationship between sex differences and job performance. In 1926 Women's Bureau investigators had found numerous instances of women's higher absenteeism and sickness rates, which increased when women worked at night. European investigations, on which many U.S. policies were based, had cited women's "lower resistance" to the strains of industry.[18]

In addition to the reproductive effects of poisons, biology had figured in the studies of fatigue and the "toxic build-up" that created "inflammatory mischief arising around the generative organs," according to Josephine Goldmark.[19] Emphasizing biology also implied a reliance on scientific evidence, which helped grant legitimacy to a protectionist stance in an era of professionalization. The over-reliance on biology, however, worked against protectionist arguments because, if biological differences between men and women became seen as legitimate, other distinctions, such as those among women and between individuals, also might seem plausible. Emphasizing biological differences reduced the significance of broad social differences, which had contributed a major support block for protective labor legislation. Biological difference was a double-edged sword: each side feared that recognizing it would support the other's position.

By publicly ignoring the distinction between hours legislation, based largely on social differences between men and women, and legislation that prohibited women from working with certain materials, rooted in biological scientific evidence, feminists on both sides failed to achieve any real common ground. Pro-ERA feminists faced a losing battle on two fronts. First, as long as working women continued to do two jobs, and feminists did not challenge the underlying social structure that charged women with home responsibilities, hours restrictions would continue to matter to many married working women. Second, equal rights feminists failed to distinguish between jobs that posed unique physiological dangers to women and work that might have been successfully challenged based on nonsexual characteristics. This lack of distinction also limited serious attempts to alter laws on a case-by-case basis.

Protectionist feminists had also ignored distinctions between restricting hours and prohibiting exposure to poisons and had kept the spotlight on the most visible aspect of protective legislation—hours. While they allied successfully with labor unions during the New Deal years to ensure passage of hours and minimum wage legislation, these feminists' failure to distinguish between married and single working women limited their ability to speak to the variety of women's concerns about health, about children, about adequate wages, and about educational opportunities. Feminists on both sides continued to speak past each other until the 1960s.[20]

In the 1920s Hamilton had argued that both groups of feminists agreed on the ends of the ERA, but not the means. She, along with some other protectionists, had favored the repeal or alteration, "one by one [of] the laws that now hamper women or work injustice to them."[21] Protectionists adopted a collective approach. They had faith that improved conditions for *some* working women would best come about by considering *all* women as a separate category of workers, and that this would overcome what they viewed as individual women's political and economic weaknesses relative to men's in the workplace. Conversely,

ERA supporters, by basing their position on women's similarities to men, had argued that recognizing women's individual strengths and opportunities would increase only after the passage of the ERA. "The battle," wrote one feminist, would then appropriately "center on the point of woman's right to sell her labor on the same terms as men."[22]

These different approaches to feminism—one based on a collective recognition of gender roles and the other on individualism—in many ways resembled the differences between old and new medicine during the first thirty years of the twentieth century. Old medicine relied on holistic explanations for illness, as physicians, believing that all parts of the body were inextricably linked, treated the whole patient. The advance of new medicine presaged a much more specific approach to disease, one that treated the discrete body parts affected by germs. Translated into social policy, germ theory tended to promote individuals' responsibility for personal health. Previously, when good human health had appeared to have resulted from living in a healthy environment, collective action and responsibility for good health had seemed more appropriate.[23]

In the language of medicine, then, the ERA promoted an individualist approach to health in the workplace. In 1924 Doris Stevens had urged that specific, individual characteristics be used in determining employment suitability. Protective legislation penalized "*all* women because *some* women are morally frail and physically weak [emphases added]," she wrote, and "natural fitness, not 'protection,' will determine the extent of competition."[24] Protectionist arguments, however, were informed by a more holistic understanding of health. They recognized the influences of the social environment, such as women's responsibilities at home and generally poor living conditions. Like the tension between old and new medicine in occupational health policies, opposing positions on the ERA suggest that while interest in the strengths and talents of individual women had gained favor among some feminists, an understanding of the social aspects of working women's lives had not disappeared in the 1920s and 1930s.

Hamilton was a link between these contrasting intellectual and political positions on feminism, medicine, labor legislation, and public health. A feminist, she recognized the unequal economic position of women in the workplace and had suffered discrimination herself as a female physician in a male-dominated profession. Hamilton had witnessed paternalism from employers who treated women workers as poor victims—even as they ignored much more horrendous conditions for their male employees—and acknowledged the unfairness of societal (and male) expectations that working women also perform all household and child care duties. Perhaps most important, she had pointed out the selectivity of protective laws, instances where men benefited from laws that "protected" women out of certain trades. She saw the incongruity of using "physically hazardous" as an exclusionary qualification for women, observing that if society truly cared about such dangers, "we should not have tens of thousands [of women] scrubbing floors or working over the washtub."[25]

Hamilton's medical philosophy likewise straddled two sets of ideas. Despite her medical training and her ability to diagnose based on very specific blood and tissue changes, Hamilton's thinking had continued to be informed by old medicine. Her studies for the government had taken her into workers' homes, where she could not help but notice the relationship between poor health and poverty. In her autobiography she described Appalachian towns set up to house smelting plant workers and their families. The setting was depressing, the people poor: "They [workers and housing] were full of malaria, hookworm, and silica dust . . . to say nothing of lead." It was easy enough, she recalled, "to pick up cases of lead poisoning, of anemia and emaciation, of palsy, and plenty of histories of lead colic."[26]

As a scientist, however, Hamilton sought answers for specific problems in the workplace, examining the processes and materials used in manufacturing. Following Hamilton during a 1927 tour of a storage battery plant, a witness might have observed her examining blueprints, inspecting ventilation hoods, recording and pointing out specific dust hazards, instructing plant supervisors on the need for adequate sanitation facilities, consulting with the medical director, and analyzing blood samples taken from workers. She then observed what seemed to be several causes and effects supported by her laboratory research: lifting heavy objects and visible muscle strain; lead dust and paralysis; the presence of benzene and excessive bleeding; exposure to carbon disulfide and insanity. Incorporating the theoretical into the observable, Hamilton's actions revealed her reliance on environmental causes of ill health as well as their biological origins. In the course of her work, which largely focused on male workers, she had discovered, of course, that many of these hazards harmed men and women equally. She also paid attention to hazards that affected women disproportionately because they occurred in female-dominated industries.[27]

Hamilton often acted as a brake on more activist approaches to occupational health. In 1924 she supported the National Consumers' League general secretary, Florence Kelley, in the league's efforts to fund research on industrial benzene, but she warned Kelley to be careful until they became "better informed about certain puzzling features of benzene poisoning" that had begun to appear in the female-dominated can industry. Hamilton the social reformer desired action; Hamilton the scientist sought accuracy.[28]

She thus employed both environmental and individualist practices in helping industrial physicians and employers to improve the workplace and to separate occupational and non-occupational causes of disease in the industrial environment. Employers wanted to define such diseases narrowly, but Hamilton preferred to change the environment first rather than "fixing" workers after they got sick.[29]

Hamilton's professional experiences and her feminism molded her position on protective labor legislation. On the one hand, given her medical expertise, it is not surprising that she differentiated between women's social and biological roles, developing a somewhat more complex view of protective labor legislation than was the norm. On the other hand, her understanding of women's social roles prompted her to invoke the premises of old medicine in her support for protective legislation. Women worked because they had to, she believed, but that did not relieve them of household responsibilities after the factory shift was over. In 1925 Hamilton speculated that men might some day feel compelled to help out with the household duties, but until and unless that day arrived, "the working mother . . . handicapped by her own nature," would benefit from laws that limited the number of hours she could work in the factory or in business.[30]

Hamilton's work as a factory investigator provided a very clear environmental rationale for protective laws. Poverty undermined the health of many working people with poor nutrition (even if the role of nutrition was unclear) and no access to private physicians. Poverty also made it more likely that more than one family member would work for wages. Lack of skills and education often translated into low wages and little chance for advancement. Women of all ages experienced this cycle of poverty, wage work, and poor health. In candy factories Hamilton and others had found young girls working with "unmistakable signs of malnutrition and [the] lack of care that comes with poverty-stricken backgrounds." These workers tended to be "undersized, white-faced girl[s] who looked younger than their age." Low wages scarcely improved their health.[31] Working mothers with young children suffered more than other women, according to most factory investigators, because they tended to work the night shift, get little sleep during the day, receive low pay because of inferior work, and develop serious health problems.[32]

Pregnant women who worked suffered from additional fatigue and also exposed their unborn children to the unhealthy work environment. Sickly children grew up to breed yet more unhealthy children, eventually creating a drain on the community. Like many Progressive Era reformers and physicians, Hamilton was influenced by theories favoring the inheritability of characteristics acquired in the environment. She believed that the health of mothers affected infant mortality and morbidity. Having observed pediatricians' efforts to improve maternal and infant health, Hamilton worried about the future of a race that was increasingly the progeny of sickly, overfatigued industrial workers.[33]

Hamilton's medical background also encouraged her to consider biological distinctions between men and women. Unlike most protectionists, she believed that such differences deserved significant attention in determining workplace regulations. As early as 1917 she had asserted that only jobs with hazards that affected women more seriously than men should be closed to women. Examples included jobs involving exposure to poisons like lead and jobs that entailed lifting heavy weights, both conditions that adversely affected women's reproductive health.

Lead poisoning created blood changes that damaged organs and could also cause paralysis. By 1917 Hamilton knew that lead affected men's reproductive functions, but she expressed more concern about women exposed to lead throughout pregnancy. Such exposure increased the chances that children would become "leaded," because lead "circulating in the blood of the mother" could be passed on to the fetus. Instead of advocating the complete prohibition of women in the lead industries, however, Hamilton carefully defined specific jobs in various lead industries where, if employers and workers observed proper precautions and sanitation, women could safely work. Since, despite such precautions, exposure might still occur, hours restrictions in these plants remained vital: Hamilton believed that fatigue increased susceptibility to lead poisoning. Given sufficient time away from the plant, the body would eliminate absorbed lead on its own. But policymakers and employers from the 1910s through the 1940s paid little attention to Hamilton's distinctions.[34]

Hamilton's reliance on biology and her social awareness guided her attitudes about workplace regulations for men and for women. Much of her work revolved around industries whose workforce was predominantly male. In these industries reproductive function seemed to have received little if any attention, although she noted those where it had. The important point is that she did not consider women workers necessarily more victimized by industrial conditions than male workers. For example, throughout her involvement with radium dial painters in New Jersey in the 1920s, there is no evidence that she portrayed the women who contracted radium poisoning as especially deserving of sympathy because they were women. During and after the lawsuits and publicity against United States Radium Corporation, Hamilton did not advocate the elimination of women from the radium industry, but instead used these cases of radium poisoning to press for workers' compensation coverage of occupational diseases in New Jersey.[35]

Hamilton's perspectives on feminism, women's health, and protective legislation were also shaped by her involvement in public health activities. In the Progressive Era, settlement houses like Hull House in Chicago had provided a variety of free services for city residents for a specified period of time, hoping that the value of such services would be recognized—and subsequently offered—by the city. Settlement-house residents like Hamilton frequently became involved with a number of ongoing maternal health services such as well-baby clinics, sanitary milk stations, and birth control services.[36]

The benefits of public health measures were not always immediately apparent to their beneficiaries, however. Debates over the mandatory reporting of tuberculosis, the implementation of compulsory vaccination, and efforts to stop the spread of polio in pre-vaccine days, for instance, all highlighted the trade-offs associated with public health measures. Opponents of such measures had argued that public health laws left risky behavior unaltered while unfairly restricting the rights of individuals who acted responsibly. These opponents promoted education, not coercion, because in their view coercion alone did little to promote real change in behavior and instill personal responsibility. Public health proponents agreed but argued that restrictions effectively protected both less responsible individuals and the public at large.[37]

The protective labor legislation of the early twentieth century could be described as a form of public health; measures hindered individual employment rights, but they ostensibly improved society by coercing women and employers to comply with laws designed to keep the female working population healthy. The point of such public health laws was that those both disadvantaged and unaffected by such laws would presumably go along with them because they believed that public health laws promoted the greater good. Hamilton herself believed "modern sanitary progress" relied on public acceptance of the "burdens of cooperation" that public health laws might require of the citizenry.[38]

Hamilton adapted this public health approach to protective labor legislation. She had always recognized that protective laws were selective, inappropriately excluding domestic and agricultural workers, for example. She had also noted that some women workers, especially printers, would be hampered by a law that restricted women from working nights, but she had resolved both situations for herself by considering the greater good of all women and of society, again relying on a categorical definition of womanhood. Her approach was two-pronged, providing both practical, short-term relief of the problem of women's overwork and long-term education and prevention. Short-term relief took the form of hours, night work, and lifting restrictions, as well as some completely prohibitory legislation.

Hamilton's long-term goals included changing the social structure so that husbands helped with housework; economic incentives to get employers to safeguard all workers' health; and educational efforts to improve personal health standards. Some activists viewed protective laws as temporary expedients until economic conditions had improved sufficiently so that no women worked.

Long-term preventive measures also included epidemiological and scientific studies to define specific occupational diseases, which had become increasingly important as more states adopted workers' compensation for work-related illnesses. Another long-term goal that Hamilton and many other protectionists sought was the extension of protective legislation to all workers. From its inception in 1920, the U.S. Women's Bureau, an advocate for working-class women, had viewed such legislation as an entering wedge, laws that would eventually be expanded to cover male wage-earners. The Women's Bureau declared that most of its employment recommendations in cases where legislation did not yet exist should "apply fully as strongly to men as to women." In the meantime, wrote Hamilton, it was "better not to give up the ferry-boat before the bridge [was] built."[39]

Because Hamilton believed that protective laws provided a means to obtaining a safer workplace for all, she opposed the ERA, which would eliminate such legislation. Even though she supported some very specific rules that restricted women's involvement in certain work processes, she still placed all wage-earning women in one group.

Hamilton and her fellow protectionists had become state and federal bureaucrats by the 1920s and 1930s. They proceeded to institutionalize gender-based policies, as well as advocating better protection for all workers through hours legislation and workers' compensation coverage for occupational disease.[40] But despite the policymaking power of feminists who opposed the ERA, the influence of ERA supporters should not be underestimated. Arguments that emerged over the ERA in the 1920s also affected the development of occupational safety and health practices. The National Woman's Party had continuously pressed policymakers to be very careful in establishing restrictive employment standards. For their part, protectionist bureaucrats, mindful of the National Woman's Party, crafted policy statements regarding employment and health very specifically. The National Woman's Party held these bureaucrats' feet to the fire, making sure that any proposals restricting women workers remained as limited as possible.

Hamilton continued to rely on new knowledge about industrial poisons. By the 1940s she confided to the new Women's Bureau director, Frieda Miller, that some of the prohibitory legislation in the states was absurd. Hamilton accused states of ignoring dangerous poisons and placing too much emphasis on "unimportant ones." With an eye to political winds, she also wondered if such behavior played "right into the hands of the Woman's Party." During World War II, when asked for her comments on a proposed Women's Bureau bulletin, she opposed many of the items on the list of industrial poisons from which "women should be especially protected," on the grounds that most of the materials, including silica, arsenic, mercury, and TNT, were not especially harmful to women. Based on present medical knowledge and authority, she said, only lead and benzene should be on the list.[41]

Despite private doubts about the efficacy of some protective legislation, Hamilton accepted the presidency of the National Consumers' League in 1944 and, at the age of seventy-five, became head of the most vocal national organization opposing the ERA. As president (the duties of which she agreed to perform only on the condition that they did not require "active participation") Hamilton acceded to the general secretary's request to produce an article stating why she was opposed to the ERA. The league hoped that Hamilton's status would blunt the impact of the entrance of a potent new ally into the ERA battle, the American Medical Women's Association.[42]

The article appeared in *Ladies' Home Journal* in July 1945. While Hamilton publicly supported new concerns that had arisen about the ERA's possible negative effect on alimony, her strongest stated reasons for opposing the amendment had to do with the elimination of protective labor laws. Men and women are different, she argued, and although these differences had been exaggerated in the past, "Women still have to bear the babies." And women, she continued, "still ought to rear the children."[43]

Making careful use of her statistics, however, she used age as a category as well as gender, noting that most working women were young. Younger people were more susceptible to poison and fatigue, she wrote, and took less care of their own health. Younger workers also drew lower wages. Older women risked harm because of double duty. Hamilton supported protective laws as an expedient until all workers were protected, something not yet possible. The best method for achieving protection for all workers was through state, not federal, action, removing barriers to women's full and equal participation in the workforce one by one. Predicting a long road ahead, she expressed some skepticism that even that method would prove useful. She believed that custom and tradition, not law, often determined employment policies when it came to gender.[44]

Although Hamilton's article did not address the overuse of prohibitory legislation, she did begin to question it publicly in other forums. In a speech before the American Industrial Hygiene Association in 1948, she refuted the conventional wisdom that women were more susceptible to lead poisoning than men. "Careful observation," she asserted, "has not given proof of it."[45]

By the 1940s many protective laws appeared foolish to Hamilton. It was clear that they did not accomplish their original purpose. Instead, some of them seemed to serve the needs of men seeking to protect their own jobs. These types of laws played into the hands of the National Woman's Party, which was happy to use them as examples of how the National Consumers' League's support for protective laws promoted outright discrimination against women. As a corrective Hamilton supported efforts in Ohio to keep a Toledo company from prohibiting women from working at grinding and buffing jobs. The legislative committee of the Ohio Consumers' League felt that male employers inappropriately used state labor laws to freeze out women workers after the war. The only excuse for such a law, said Hamilton, would be where no protection against dust existed, and she believed that the Ohio law provided "very complete protection against the dust raised in grinding."[46]

After writing the *Ladies' Home Journal* article, she became intrigued by the arguments of a recent National Woman's Party convert, Florence Kitchelt, who in a letter suggested that the ERA would not eliminate protective legislation. After receiving what she considered inadequate refutation of Kitchelt's position from both the former Women's Bureau director Mary Anderson and the League of Women Voters, Hamilton sought out the Consumers' League's general secretary, Elizabeth Magee, who likewise urged her to ignore this latest "ploy" of the National Woman's Party to garner support for its position. But Hamilton did not ignore it, and in 1952, apparently without letting the league know ahead of time, she allowed Kitchelt to publish a statement announcing Hamilton's repudiation of her opposition to the ERA.[47]

Why did she change her mind? Many of the social conditions that Hamilton had always hoped for—the use of protective legislation as a wedge for achieving better conditions for all workers; decreased paternalism on the part of employers who saw that, given the chance, women did well in many jobs; passage of workers' compensation laws for occupational diseases in many states; and recognition by many that women should get help in performing their double duty—had begun to emerge. Hamilton also believed that health and safety had become sufficiently important to unions, to the state, and to employers, especially with the passage of workers' compensation legislation. Also, after World War II, many people had trouble making a convincing argument that women lacked the physical fitness needed for work in industry and were unable to balance household and wage work. Finally, Hamilton supported Eleanor Roosevelt's belief that U.S. support for equal rights for women would give the nation more credibility in the United Nations' newly created Commission on Human Rights.[48]

With good evidence for many wage-earning women's improved social conditions, Hamilton's expertise and interest in specific biological and scientific aspects of occupational health became more visible. In the forty years since she had begun investigating the "dangerous trades," hygienic conditions in plants had noticeably improved. Medical knowledge had increased the ability of employers to keep workers healthy and to open up opportunities for women in many plants. By 1948, for example, Hamilton had reversed a long-held belief, stating that she was no longer strongly convinced that benzene was more dangerous to "menstruating girls than to young men." Protective laws seemed to have served their purpose in providing short-term, practical relief while reformers worked for longer-term changes in behavior and attitudes. As public health measures, many of these laws and policies had become institutionalized in other parts of government, in industry, and in labor relations. Moreover, the tremendous variety of working women's circumstances by the early 1950s made many protective laws too sweeping.[49]

In 1953, responding to Hamilton's change in position, Magee apparently persuaded her that hours laws and minimum wage laws in most states would be jeopardized by the passage of the ERA because only a few applied to both men and women. Hamilton apologized to Magee for her "ill-considered action," but Magee, to the great consternation of other Consumers' League members, chose not to demand a more public clarification from Hamilton, which is surprising given the publicity that the National Woman's Party had devoted to her change of heart. Instead Magee circulated copies of Hamilton's letter to members of the league. It appears that although Hamilton was willing to admit to an error with respect to special legislation, she gave no indication of reconsidering her decision about the ERA. She continued to support both the U.N. Commission on Human Rights and revisions in alimony and child support laws, which she felt were "unfairly weighted in favor of women and should be changed to conform to modern ideas." Although she did not mention health or medical issues, Hamilton was clearly thinking beyond simple, categorical definitions of "womanhood" and "motherhood," acknowledging the existence of a more complicated gender structure marked by individual differences among women.[50]

The Women's Bureau followed the lead of Roosevelt and Hamilton. In 1954 the official newsletter of the National Woman's Party gleefully reported that the bureau would no longer take a position against the ERA. The Women's Bureau's noncommittal position, according to the historian Alice Kessler-Harris, reflected the improved position of wage-earning women's lives and pushed the bureau into a more activist position for women's occupational and economic advancement.[51]

The ERA debate functioned as a catalyst and a dialectic, forcing feminists on both sides to engage in a continual assessment and sharpening of their proposals on women's workplace health. Each interaction resulted in incremental changes, eventually creating space for more complex views of womanhood and a more diverse workplace. Hamilton provided a bridge between those who organized around a categorical, holistic definition of motherhood ("social" motherhood) and those who envisioned a more diverse, yet more individualistic and narrowly defined role ("biological" motherhood). While working conditions improved for both men and women, and more women entered nontraditional jobs, the consequences of treating women as individuals undermined traditional strategies—with the unexpected result of achieving change on behalf of all women.

6

Women and the Environment: *"The Pathology and Hygiene of Housework"*

In the 1960s the term "environmentalism" still had multiple meanings. Many agendas surfaced that eventually provided a suitable public forum for a distinctly gendered activism around workplace health in the 1970s. Issues raised by women workers with respect to their health and safety needs during World War II influenced the postwar workplace. Some workplace policies were consistent with trends established in the 1930s. Many industrial physicians stressed the need to consider the worker as more than a worker. Like employers' efforts in the 1920s to attribute workplace ailments to personal behavior, policies in the 1950s paid more attention to workers' psychological and mental health than to their physical health. "Company after company," according to an oil company staff physician, "has come to realize that psychosomatic ailments can be as disabling as physical accidents, so they've called in psychologists to set up human relations programs."[1]

While some of this can accurately be attributed to increased general public interest in psychological behavior, the experiences of working mothers during World War II exposed a significant link between occupational and non-occupational health. Employers during the war had tried to assimilate women into the workplace as quickly as possible by making changes necessary to accommodate physical differences from men and by providing women with the same protective gear and rules as men. When absenteeism rates continued to be higher among women workers, employers had been forced to acknowledge that gender-specific, non-occupational factors influenced workplace health. In wartime's tight labor market, employers began hiring female counselors to do what was necessary to reduce female absenteeism, but after the war, many of these counselors were laid off. The notion that a worker's home life affected productivity on the job, however, remained. In the 1920s and 1930s many employers had sought to link workers' non-occupational behavior to workplace health problems. In the 1950s employers established company-sponsored programs for any number of ills.[2]

Employers also expanded the use of pre-employment physical examinations. Pre-employment exams had helped employers place women in war-related industrial jobs during World War II, but they also allowed industrial physicians to screen for any predispositions that might be exacerbated by certain kinds of employment. "Less time, effort and expense in training . . . will be spent," said a National Association of Manufacturers director before a 1956 audience, "if it is discovered before employment or not long afterwards that the employee's physical capacities are not equal to the physical demands of the job." Workers, however, acquiesced only reluctantly to such examinations, as evidenced by a lengthy description of how to outsmart such workers. "History-taking is useless," Dr. Katharine Sturgis wrote in 1956, "since, in the desire to obtain work, most applicants deny the presence of symptoms or a history of major illness." She recommended more "discreet" methods of detecting respiratory diseases in applicants, such as implying to would-be employees that the X-ray had already indicated an abnormality. Under these circumstances, she advised, "the applicant usually tells the truth, often having rightly or wrongly given up hope of securing the job and [being] seriously interested in obtaining information pertinent to his health."[3]

Sturgis, chair of the Preventive Medicine Department at the Woman's Medical College of Pennsylvania, also promoted the study of workers because they were relatively stable populations, which were preferable in prospective studies (those that followed subjects over a period of time, noting changes). Sturgis supervised such research among male workers throughout the 1950s and early 1960s, testing for early signs of lung cancer. She used her data to link lung cancer with cigarette smoking among workers, not with workplace hazards. Similarly, the Uterine Cancer Cytology Research Project in 1957 recorded the incidence of uterine cancer among women in industry in the Philadelphia area. While these data recorded where these women worked, it is clear that members of the research team used this cohort of women to determine the incidence of uterine cancer among women throughout the region, not correlating workplace with illness. Using employees at the workplace was far simpler logistically than following up on women in their homes.[4]

Efforts to understand workers' lifestyles, either through in-plant health programs or through the study of workers as a microcosm of the larger community, represent a broader shift in responsibility for workplace health from government to private industry in the 1950s. David Rosner and Gerald Markowitz have noted a decline in government interest in occupational health and safety in the postwar period along with a concomitant rise in the authority of the scientific community. Both trends resulted in greater control by industry. Specialists in industrial medicine increasingly rejected what they called the "overdiagnosis" of industrial disease by local physicians and argued that more responsibility be placed with industrial physicians. While this has sometimes been viewed as a case of the fox guarding the henhouse, Rosner and Markowitz and others note that, in the late 1940s and the 1950s, the legitimacy of the laboratory over the more subjective diagnosis of the clinician was seldom challenged.[5]

Government yielded to industry and insurance companies in the wake of increased workers' compensation coverage for occupational disease, which created an additional impetus for more precise diagnosis. Some physicians also faulted government regulations for not adequately protecting workers. After examining Massachusetts regulations governing the employment of women, Alice Hamilton charged that the regulations inappropriately excluded women from some safer jobs while they ignored the more dangerous ones. For instance, Massachusetts Department of Labor and Industry rules required the installation of a number of "suitable partitions" and self-closing doors in the core-making rooms of foundries before women could be employed in them, a regulation she found foolish.[6]

Hamilton likewise questioned the efficacy of an Ohio regulation that prohibited the employment of women in any grinding and polishing operations and persuaded women workers to oppose the regulations. "If the exhausts on the machines are according to the legal requirements," argued Hamilton, there was no reason to exclude women from these jobs. "Women," she wrote, "are no more susceptible to [the dusts created by grinding steel, copper and brass] . . . and to dust of the abrasives than men are."[7]

By the end of World War II, state protective labor laws, which had been lifted during the war, seemed glaringly discriminatory and arbitrary to many. The ERA supporter Nora Stanton Barney (a granddaughter of Elizabeth Cady Stanton) remarked that a woman could legally carry seventy-five pounds in Massachusetts, but in California, she would be prohibited from carrying more than ten pounds up a flight of stairs. Aside from the dubious assertion that women in California were somehow weaker than their sisters in New England, Barney wondered how mothers were to carry their children in California. Dismissing claims that medical science supported weight restrictions, she also alleged that "what was considered injurious to the health of women has differed from generation to generation," and had been controlled by prejudice, not science.[8]

Government advocacy for working women also started to crumble at the federal level. The Women's Bureau, solidly grounded in protectionist tradition from its inception in 1920 through World War II, shifted gears after the war. Alice Kessler-Harris has argued that New Deal labor policies improving health conditions for industrial workers of both sexes, as well as the spread of trade unionism to many working women, undermined arguments for special protection. By the early 1950s the Women's Bureau had consciously but slowly shifted its advocacy role from one of improving the working conditions of women because they needed special protection to one of promoting equal opportunities for women based on their rights as members of a free-market economy. The Women's Bureau virtually stopped studying working-class women and began to focus more on professional women.[9]

Until the 1950s the bureau had consistently favored sex-based protective labor legislation as an expedient, pending the proper protection of all workers. Even so, by the early 1940s, some bureau researchers had recognized the limitations of the policy. Few states even had specific legislation, and the bureau argued that none of the general provisions that several states had laid down about working women's "health and morals" had "ever been applied to the prevention of occupational disease." Above all, it favored broader workers' compensation coverage for occupational diseases. The bureau had little faith in the efficacy of compulsory reporting of occupational diseases by physicians. In 1934 twenty states had required such reporting either to state labor boards or to public health departments, but there seems to be little evidence that the reports resulted in any changes at the state level.[10]

The Women's Bureau's advocacy on behalf of industrial health declined when it finally dropped its opposition to the ERA in 1954, and this weakening of the bureau's efforts helped industry attain more control over determining workplace health standards.[11] Nevertheless, the bureau's impact should not be underestimated; in many ways its ideas allowed for the numerous shifts that occurred during the 1950s, 1960s, and 1970s. Legitimizing the study of workplace hazards that disproportionately affected women provided a model for a medical study of housework in 1950. The bureau's insistence on linking household and workplace resonated with activists in the 1960s who wanted to curb environmental damage done by industry. And the serious attention given working women by the bureau buttressed calls for gender equality in the 1960s and 1970s.

When the Medical Women's International Association (MWIA) met in Philadelphia in 1950, the planning committee had been organizing a "pathology and hygiene of housework" scientific session for nearly two years. The idea for the session grew out of a 1948 MWIA council discussion of the medical problems associated with housework. Charged with developing methods of improving "conditions for the housewife," the council's co-chairs, Dr. Maria Teresa Casassa of Italy and Dr. Gerda Seidelin Wegener of Denmark, wrote up a questionnaire and divided it into four parts: diseases of household workers, hours and working conditions, availability and quality of training in household skills, and legislation governing "domestic workers."[12]

In designing this questionnaire, the two physicians tried hard to apply traditional industrial workplace characteristics to housework. Under part 2, for instance ("Hygiene"), they asked for information about hours, sanitary facilities, day care, and vacation time. Under "Diseases" they listed several conditions known to be common to domestic workers—among them varicose veins, dermatoses, and muscular diseases. They resisted attempts by the MWIA's executive committee to change the name of the session to give more emphasis to "the health of the housewife." Wegener and Casassa both insisted that focusing on the tasks associated with housework rather than on the life of the housewife would provide more reliable, consistent, and tenable results. "If we go from house-work to house-wife," wrote Wegener, "the subject to me seems endless and impossible to limit."[13]

Women physicians applied traditional occupational safety and health standards to describe a workplace with which industrial physicians and safety engineers were not familiar. The home, with its irregular work hours, no workers' compensation, and unpredictable job changes, was a workplace that did not yield easy comparisons. Nevertheless, many concluded that houses and tasks could be designed to reduce wear and tear on the housewife, allowing her to devote time to the more creative aspects of her life.

For the most part organizers maintained the industrial model in their questionnaire, but some modifications had to be made to accommodate the international nature of their organization. The MWIA's secretary general, Dr. Germaine Montreuil-Straus, reminded Casassa and Wegener to distinguish between the "townswoman" and the "peasant" in considering the organization of housework. Casassa and Wegener also agreed to include "the carrying of water" in their list of household tasks. Indeed, the tasks they proposed to study applied equally to housewives and domestics, although respondents largely focused on wives who performed housework.[14]

The committee compiled replies from fifteen nations and publicized them at the September 1950 meeting, held at Woman's Medical College in Philadelphia. Housework per se caused no pathology—the tasks themselves were "extremely important" to society—but the working conditions under which it was performed needed improvement: long working hours, inadequate housing, few labor-saving appliances. Reports from most countries indicated that female wage workers, peasants, and full-time housewives worldwide wanted a different work environment—better equipment, better training, and improved working and living conditions, all of which would reduce the major symptoms of housework: overwork and fatigue. Those attending the conference visited a downtown model home outfitted with the latest household appliances, including a "work simplification" kitchen designed by the New York Heart Association with the help of an industrial efficiency expert, Lillian Gilbreth.[15]

Respondents also sought social recognition for housework. Many physicians observed that society attached value only to wage work. Consequently many members and presenters at this session believed that the workplace needed to be reconfigured structurally and socially—with new housework rules that required help from all family members, furniture and household appliances built to avoid excessive bending or reaching, and appreciation of the "10- to 20-hour day profession" of housework. Despite popular 1950s images celebrating domesticity, the MWIA's Sixth Congress called on the authority of the medical profession to "solve the manifold problems associated with 'occupation—housewife.'"[16]

In contrast to her European and Asian colleagues, a U.S. presenter at the conference applied a different industrial model to housework, one that more closely resembled efforts by industrial physicians in the 1950s. Using the scientific session as a forum to tout U.S. economic superiority, and in some ways anticipating the 1959 Nixon-Khrushchev "kitchen debate," Dr. Audrey Bobb of New York University Medical School argued that the biggest problem of the U.S. housewife was her "values." Instead of changing the workplace, which, according to Bobb, had "superior working conditions, food, and mechanical help," U.S. women needed to learn how to manage their time better. "Old-fashioned exercise" and "sensible shoes" would relieve U.S. housewives of any fatigue they complained of. "What is she doing with all the leisure time that the machine is giving her?" asked Bobb. "What inner resources is she developing? What value is she living by?" The message was similar to one promoted by U.S. industry: the personal habits of the worker, not the workplace environment, were most often responsible for poor workplace health. Consistent with another common employer strategy aimed at changing the worker, Bobb also prevailed upon women to see this work as "completely rewarding and satisfying."[17]

Most of those attending the congress, however, recognized the need for changes in the work environment, not the workers' attitudes. The MWIA's solutions reflected more modern assumptions about women and work. Unlike the previous generation, which had viewed women's household roles as antithetical to industrial work, these women physicians justified women's household duties in the context of modern industrial health and safety, separating housework from child-rearing. And in applying workplace standards to what had been considered a private domain, they helped legitimize an increasingly common public image in the 1950s, the married working woman. Moreover, these women physicians did not emphasize women's inherent weakness relative to men. Informed by different assumptions about women, they argued that the work of housework need not be all-consuming. Ultimately, their view of the role of the housewife, which encompassed both childbearing and child-rearing, went beyond notions of housework. They clearly favored separating the work from the wife, suggesting a divisibility and a specialization of tasks associated with motherhood.

In sharp contrast to arguments made in favor of sex-based protective labor legislation a generation earlier, the medical evidence offered in support of easing housework's more fatiguing tasks did not suggest that the workplace was dangerous for women. Instead, women physicians considered these women real workers, deserving of any and all protections provided to wage workers.

Another indication of the continuing links between home and workplace can be seen in postwar environmental activism. Consumers' Leagues across the country began to focus less on the industrial environment in the 1950s. While they remained committed to protective labor legislation for women, as well as to more general legislation regulating the workplace, many state organizations turned to labor issues specific to their region. The Connecticut and New Jersey leagues, for instance, devoted time and resources to the working conditions of migrant workers within their borders, especially the revival of child labor in agricultural labor camps.[18]

This shift away from environmental issues was short-lived, however. In the late 1950s, the New Jersey league asked the national office for help in producing and distributing to the public useful information about radiation hazards. While there were no nuclear industries in New Jersey at the time, the league's state secretary, Susanna Zwemer, recalled the organization's role in exposing hazards in the radium dial painting industry in the 1920s. She began a campaign for national regulations to ensure the health and safety of the growing numbers of workers using radioactive materials.[19]

Zwemer's activism, which was reminiscent of earlier Consumers' League work on behalf of safe working conditions, went beyond considering ill effects on workers. Effective preventive measures for workers were important, she wrote in 1958, but "the problem of radiation exposure affects all the population—it can be just as deadly outside the walls of the factory or the hospital."[20]

The National Consumers' League and many other labor and health organizations believed workers' compensation legislation to be inadequate because of radiation poisoning's long latency period, which often exhausted the statute of limitations set by many compensation laws. Responding to Hamilton's fears that proper safeguards in individual states would not provide the expertise necessary in this new and constantly changing industry, the National Consumers' League called for uniform federal standards in maintaining radiation safety. "The protection of workers, their families, and their communities from dangerous radiation exposure" was the most important issue of the period, according to the National Consumers' League board of directors in 1959.[21]

Claudia Clark has characterized the actions of the Consumers' Leagues with respect to radiation safety as an example of the continuing vitality of Progressive Era reform organizations.[22] The concern about radiation hazards also reflects a continuity of environmentalism, as the concept was envisioned by the leagues' turn-of-the-century founders. Their belief that the workplace was hazardous to the health of families was reflected in the actions of their daughters, who focused on changing the workplace rather than the worker or the home. In 1959 the National Consumers' League general secretary, Vera Mayer, compared the need for federal regulations to the ubiquitous nature of radiation exposure itself:

> Just as this problem transcends national boundaries, so does the radiation exposure of workers transcend the factory walls. I do not at this stage see any way of separating out the worker in a factory utilizing radioactive isotopes from a variety of circumstances that effect [sic] the worker as a member of the community. Take the case of a worker in a plant which uses radioactive isotopes for peacetime industry. This worker has had X-rays of his teeth and chest; he lives in a community whose natural rock formations may give off varying amounts of "background" radiation; he breathes air and eats food as all members of his community do which may be contaminated to varying degrees with fallout particles. To attempt to establish a standard of "permissible radiation exposure" for this worker only in terms of the exposure level in the plant would represent a very artificial treatment of the problem. Indeed, I fear that such an approach might very well be dangerous since the worker would be lulled into a feeling of security when actually the work exposure taken together with the other types of radiation he is receiving could conceivably take him over the "permissible" level.[23]

By the late 1950s many citizens had become skeptical of industry's ability to regulate itself, and there were successful attempts to separate the regulatory from the promotional aspects of the nuclear industry in these years. Radiation, however, was not the only hazard that crossed factory walls. As if to acknowledge this changing relationship between the workplace, the household, and the community, industrial health had been transformed first to "occupational health" and then, by the 1960s, to environmental health. Harriet L. Hardy, a physician with the Massachusetts Division of Industrial Hygiene, attributed the first shift to an acknowledgment of health hazards in a wide variety of occupations. In explaining the second, a University of California public health physician de-emphasized scientific advances in favor of a growing social awareness of environmental and community stresses on the body.[24]

Such awareness had serious implications for the workplace, but not all groups responded with the alacrity of the Consumers' League of New Jersey. Many in the medical profession interpreted this environmental license in ways that sometimes resembled the by now common strategies of employers to reduce industrial responsibility for maintaining a healthy environment.

A "killer smog" that had descended on the steel town of Donora, Pennsylvania, in 1948 awakened the public to the postwar reality of air pollution, already visible in southern California. By 1960 numerous instances of chronic industrial air hazards had increased public awareness. And Dr. Katharine Sturgis, whose research on male workers had led her to promote antismoking measures rather than to search for industrial causes of lung cancer, exhibited a very different attitude toward industry when industrial pollution adversely affected the lungs of the surrounding community.[25]

In 1962 Sturgis, professor of preventive medicine at Woman's Medical College, was asked to investigate complaints from citizens in the town of Driftwood in northern central Pennsylvania. The Metal Wire Recovery Company had recently built a plant in the area to burn insulation off old telephone cable to recover the copper. The burning released polyvinyl chloride (PVC) into the air. With the help of Dr. Doris Freudenberg, a local physician, Sturgis interviewed sixty-two people in a house-to-house survey and found all but seven suffering from a variety of respiratory and intestinal irritations—nausea, nosebleeds, chest tightness. She also noted increased hospitalizations for cardiopulmonary failure and for asthma. Acid fumes created physical changes in the environment: poor visibility, pitting in aluminum chairs, bleached trees.[26]

Sturgis soon became aware of the economic implications of investigating a local plant in a rural area. One asymptomatic interviewee whose son and son-in-law worked at the plant believed, "If men can work and risk their lives, why should the community complain?" Another perceived the absence or presence of symptoms as being pro- or anti-industry, respectively. Sturgis supported the efforts, eventually successful, of the local ad hoc Citizens' Committee on Air Pollution to stop the burning. In contrast to Sturgis's apparent cooperation with industry officials when she had studied workers for signs of lung cancer, she was harshly critical of the Metal Wire Recovery Company, calling the owner an "unprincipled man" and a "ruthless entrepreneur" with a stronghold on local political and business leaders.[27]

In contrast to Consumers' League activists, who found the link between the health of workers and of the community critical in their efforts to change the industrial environment and create an "environmental movement," Sturgis promoted environmental health by targeting diseases caused by industrial pollution among nonworkers in the community. As in her earlier work on workers and smoking, she de-emphasized the dangers of industrial chemicals to workers at the Metal Wire Recovery Company. Sturgis, influenced by industrial physicians who tried to pin the bad health of workers on poor personal habits, seemed to view workers as capable of responsibly assuming any risks associated with their employment. At the same time she sympathized with people in the community as "innocent victims" of industrial excess. Interestingly, her view of the plight of the community was not unlike early twentieth-century perceptions of women workers: both were seen as helpless and in need of state protection from industrial excess.[28]

Sturgis's work on behalf of Driftwood's residents suggests a medical mistrust of business, but her research on workers indicates a medical mistrust of workers that may be explicable in terms of research methodology. Because using large groups of industrial workers for medical study required employers' cooperation, Sturgis and others did not necessarily rush to find causes of disease in workplace conditions. In this they perhaps suffered from impaired objectivity.

Despite the medical community's attitudes toward workers, Sturgis did help move industrial medicine beyond the boundaries of the factory, although with mixed results. In 1960 the American Medical Association's publication *Archives of Industrial Hygiene and Occupational Medicine* was foundering. Seeking to broaden its readership, the journal's board of directors changed the name to *Archives of Environmental Health* and hired Sturgis as editor. Sturgis solicited material from a variety of sources—including scientific papers from conferences as well as more general philosophical pieces from older colleagues. Within a few years, the *Archives* had become an international forum for preventive and environmental medicine.[29]

Articles in the *Archives* in the 1960s reflected the convergence of industrial, occupational, and environmental health issues. Medical professionals of various specialties sought to control this relatively new field of environmental health, but the 1962 publication of *Silent Spring* by Rachel Carson threatened to upset, or at least change, the parameters of the environmental discussion. Carson's account of the dire effects of herbicides and pesticides effectively placed the scientific explanations next to very personal relationships experienced by ordinary people in their everyday appreciation of nature.[30]

The medical profession responded in various ways. Many physicians who otherwise praised the works of Rachel Carson and Lewis Herber for popularizing important environmental issues cautioned against overemphasizing

Carson's "poetical and graphic evocation of a small town where the birds have ceased to sing" at the expense of technological progress. All technological innovations, wrote René Dubos, "are bound to upset the balance of nature. Technological progress necessarily involves dangers, and these cannot always be foreseen." Nevertheless, he continued, risks were necessary in order for "vigorous societies" to develop. He believed that the value of Carson's and Herber's books lay in providing an impetus for "better scientific knowledge of the biological effects of chemicals" and better control of natural forces.[31]

Sturgis echoed these concerns, calling for more informed scientific studies of specific hazards. Scientists, she said, "know the need for calm approaches to the gathering and evaluating of data." While she believed that industry offered a "splendid laboratory" for such study, she admitted that in some research, it was best not to alarm workers unnecessarily or prematurely.[32]

Workers, however, often expressed skepticism about expert efforts to "protect" them. "There are many thousands of chemicals used in industry," charged one health and safety activist at the International Union of Electrical Workers in the 1960s, "so many new ones . . . that even the experts don't know all the harmful ones. . . . Sometimes ones even the experts thought were safe turn out to be killers." He urged workers to trust themselves, warning, "If some of the workers' bodies react against it, it is not good."[33]

Once industrial medicine became linked with the environment, industry almost instinctively developed two responses. First, industrial leaders themselves took a very broad view. In addition to dangers caused by air and water pollution, radiation, and chemicals, the DuPont Company scientist John Zapp urged the consideration of such things as "food, clothing, shelter, light, sound, climate, heating and air-conditioning, traffic conditions, the social and political attitudes of others, conditions of urban and suburban living, the pressures of the job and home, the surrounding flora and fauna, etc." In this view, of course, industry could not be held responsible for all the ills of the environment, and it could take credit for many of the benefits of modern society. Second, employers urged reliance on scientific studies rather than legal action to pinpoint danger. Neither of these responses is particularly surprising, and both reflect employer attitudes expressed earlier in the century. Consumers took a somewhat different approach, using the ties being made between the public, industry, workers, and public space to promote widespread activism on behalf of environmental issues.[34]

7
Factories, Feminism, and Fetal Protection Policies

Environmentalism and feminism in the 1960s reflect the lingering influence of earlier generations, even as proponents responded to events in more "modern" ways. The rise of the environmentalist and women's movements seems to describe a full circle from the turn of the century, when households were threatened by industrial dangers. Instead of long hours and unsanitary working conditions endangering the health of the mothers who, in turn, risked the well-being of families, households in the 1960s were threatened by toxic substances in household products and in the air and water surrounding many industrial plants. Similarly, in considering the impact of the women's movement, it is important to recognize the continuing nature of feminist debate about women's differences from men, although in the 1970s the definition of such differences centered more tightly around biology.

Feminists and environmentalists during this period advocated changes in the environment, but their conceptions of environment differed. Feminists developed two strategies: (1) urging employers to implement policies that made women responsible for decisions regarding their own motherhood; and (2) agitating for better working conditions for all workers, because men's reproductive systems were also compromised by materials like lead. Environmentalists within the medical profession commonly spoke of the community surrounding the plant as the innocent victims of unhealthy industrial conditions. They sought to change the environment beyond the factory walls. With respect to workers, these environmentalists seemed to agree with feminists that workers should be responsible for their own behavior.

While the inclination to change the environment is clearly reminiscent of the early twentieth century, the assumptions made about workers seem quite different. Influenced by more than a hundred years of modern medical explanations for disease, reformers in the 1960s and 1970s operated within a much more reductionist set of guidelines about personal responsibility for health. For women workers, this resulted in a conundrum: if sex discrimination stops but the environment does not change, both male and female workers assume equal risk, not equal protection. This has been especially true with fetal protection. A reductionist approach to women's occupational health—pinpointing specific physiological differences between men and women—has helped women advance economically and socially in the workplace. But it is also important to recognize other, and perhaps dangerous, consequences. For instance, although most feminists hailed the 1991 U.S. Supreme Court decision prohibiting companies from imposing fetal protection policies on their fertile women workers, at least one feminist historian argued that the decision gave women the right to poison themselves—while doing little to make the workplace safer. Noting that "winning was better than losing," the historian Ruth Rosen still asserted that with this decision, the Supreme Court had "delivered equal opportunity jeopardy."[1]

The implications of this decision are rooted in the occupational health practices of the 1950s. In the 1950s women became more visible in the paid workplace, but government interest in workplace health regulation declined. As a result, industry began instituting its own sex-based labor policies, beginning with a fetal protection policy that prohibited all fertile women from working with lead. This was consistent with recommendations issued early in the century by industrial toxicologists. But industry's self-imposed policies differed from protective labor legislation in several ways.[2] First, protective labor laws were legislative acts, while fetal protection policies were employment policies, presumably agreed to as a condition of employment. More significantly, fetal protection policies construed motherhood narrowly, as a biological act. By focusing on the physiological aspects of childbearing, these policies indicate an awareness that motherhood, although historically comprising a variety of tasks, was becoming divided into several specific roles, only one of which was biological. And although both types of policies targeted women workers, the goal of fetal protection policies was to protect fetuses, not mothers.

Fetal protection policies first appeared in 1952 at General Motors, initially in its foundries and later in its manufacturing and battery plants. While General Motors claimed to have based its decision on scientific evidence, economic, sociological, and political factors with long-lasting repercussions also influenced the company's actions.[3]

European physicians began to notice lead's effects on female reproduction by the end of the nineteenth century, observing that women who worked with lead suffered more stillbirths and spontaneous abortions. Chronic lead poisoning ruptures red blood cells; this breakdown hinders the delivery of oxygen, leading to placental and fetal damage in pregnant women. Knowledge grew slowly about lead's effects on reproduction. By the 1920s physicians knew that lead was stored in the bones. The New York Bureau of Industrial Hygiene's recommended lead poisoning treatment was first a low milk diet, which would get the body to excrete lead, and then a diet high in calcium. Lead can also poison a fetus when it draws calcium from the mother's bones.[4]

Writing in 1947, Dr. Anna Baetjer reported that lead absorbed by pregnant women almost invariably risked damage or death to the fetus. On the issue of excessive exposure to lead preceding pregnancy, Baetjer, a public health scientist at Johns Hopkins University, admitted less certainty, although she did acknowledge that some authorities believed that "lead stored in the bones during exposure may be released subsequent to exposure as a result of certain metabolic conditions." She pointed out that other investigators did not believe this explanation, but she argued that lead in human tissue and body fluids "may remain high for some months following the exposure. Hence, it may be dangerous for women to be exposed to abnormally high concentrations of lead immediately preceding pregnancy."[5]

Lead's effects on fertility were less well-documented and largely observable through changes in menstruation—amenorrhea, dysmenorrhea, and menorrhagia (abnormally heavy menstrual flow). According to the scientists G. Vermande-Van Eck and J. W. Meigs, "The important change in ovarian function was a depression of estrogen effect [as well as] damage to the primordial oocytes and an inhibition of follicle development. . . . Ovulation failed to occur."[6]

Scientists knew that lead also affected the male reproductive system. French laboratory experiments at the turn of the century had indicated that lead damaged the germ cells of both men and women; the continued exposure of a woman and her developing fetus throughout her pregnancy, however, produced a blood lead level in the newborn that matched that of the mother. In any event, the most widely cited and publicized medical evidence had focused on women.[7]

General Motors relied on medical knowledge in developing its policy. The reproductive hazards of lead had been well documented in both medical and industrial literature for many years, and there was no question by the late 1930s that lead in some amount caused harm to female workers. Why, then, did General Motors choose to implement such a policy in the early 1950s?

One important economic factor was compensation as a cost of doing business. By the early postwar period, most states included occupational diseases under their workers' compensation laws.[8] Companies' insurance premiums, based on illness and injury rates peculiar to the type of industry and the typical hazards associated with it, reflected the potential level of risk to workers. If workers became disabled by a work-related injury or illness, insurance paid for medical costs and lost wages according to a schedule. While industries, insurance companies, and workers often haggled over the precise definition of particular occupational diseases, the workers' compensation system helped industries maintain predictable costs of doing business.

Workers' compensation insurance would presumably cover workers disabled because of lead poisoning, but no provision covered injuries to a developing fetus. A 1946 federal court decision opened the door for such litigation. Nearly sixty years after Oliver Wendell Holmes declared that a fetus was not a person and that its parents could therefore not sue for damages, a District of Columbia federal court distinguished between viable and nonviable fetuses. The judge permitted a suit on behalf of a child who had been injured by a physician during an emergency delivery following an automobile accident. A viable fetus, wrote the judge, was not part of the mother. Several subsequent cases in the late 1940s and early 1950s expanded this notion of fetal rights. Industry had become subject to lawsuits filed by the offspring of workers damaged because of hazards in their parents' workplace. This was the very reasoning used by Johnson Controls, a storage battery company, in defending its fetal protection policy before the U.S. Supreme Court in 1991: "The issue is protecting the health of unborn children.... At the same time, we have a legitimate position in protecting our shareholders' interest." The potential for more lawsuits reintroduced an unacceptable level of uncertainty into business costs, similar to the one that had precipitated the establishment of workers' compensation insurance.[9]

Another area of uncertainty within the realm of employer liability lay in the compensation aspects of obstetrical and gynecological problems. Interested physicians in the early 1950s uncovered very little current literature on the topic and warned their colleagues to begin paying attention to workplace hazards that might cause gynecological and obstetrical problems. The object was to determine which ones might be compensable, including exposure to poisons.[10]

General Motors' fetal protection policy, however, existed comfortably within the pro-business climate of the early 1950s. Employers rather than the state increasingly assumed control over workplace health, relying ever more on experts and extending their interest to encompass workers' non-workplace behavior. Specialists in industrial medicine increasingly rejected what they considered the overdiagnosis of industrial disease by local physicians. They argued that more responsibility needed to be placed with industrial physicians. Government yielded to industry and insurance companies in the wake of increased workers' compensation coverage for occupational disease, which created an additional impetus for more exact diagnosis.[11]

At the same time that fetal protection policies were instituted as a result of more precise evidence of physiological change, they also undercut longstanding employer habits of promoting personal responsibility through various forms of industrial welfare capitalism. The 1950s versions appeared as "human relations programs," encouraging industrial physicians to consider all aspects of a worker's life that might affect his or her health when determining susceptibility to occupational diseases and injuries, including risks to pregnancy. Fetal protection policies took away the element of personal responsibility for all fertile female workers. Both welfare capitalism and fetal protection policies alleviated the need for employers to change the workplace environment.[12]

The General Motors decision reflected broad sociological trends concerning families. These tendencies had become noticeable in the 1920s and 1930s; in the postwar period they became institutionalized. Many social workers acted on the belief that, while nearly all women possessed the biological capacity to bear children, not all were suited to raising them properly. In 1952 Ida Cannon, a longtime veteran of the Massachusetts General Hospital Medical Social Work Department, worried that children who stayed with their single mothers might be improperly "deprived of the security of legal parents and a true home" and urged adoption instead. Social workers might be able to help a single mother through pregnancy and delivery, but Cannon feared that "the problem of her future years and the life of her child" would result in an "insecure social position" that promised too much hardship for the "victim child." Fetal protection policies shifted attention and concern from mothers to unborn children, and many social workers did the same, increasingly supporting the rights of the young over those of their mothers.[13]

The decision to institute fetal protection policies in the workplace would have political ramifications in the future. In contrast to the widespread opposition to fetal protection policies espoused by feminists and other activists in the 1970s and 1980s, General Motors' 1952 action seems to have attracted little notice from workers or medical professionals, favorable or otherwise. The Women's Bureau, for example, neither supported nor opposed fetal protection policies. Instead it spent its time promoting women's opportunities in professional occupations.[14]

It is not surprising that feminists like Alice Hamilton and protectionist groups like the National Consumers' League did not criticize such policies. Hamilton had consistently supported the employment of more women in industrial jobs, but she had also supported excluding women from jobs that posed dangers to healthy pregnancies. As late as 1948 she continued to assert that, despite great improvements in industrial working conditions, some jobs exposed workers to lead in large enough quantities to be too hazardous to women of childbearing age. The National Consumers' League used the issue of biological difference as a visible manifestation of the need for special protection.[15]

The lack of criticism from the most vocal supporter of the newly revived Equal Rights Amendment is more puzzling. The National Woman's Party had consistently viewed sex discrimination based on medical evidence with suspicion, arguing instead that a father's health at the time of conception was as important as a mother's. Sometimes the state of the man's health was even more critical. One of the party's postwar promotional pamphlets cited Women's Bureau research during the war, which indicated that men were "rendered sterile [by ionizing radiation] in half the time" that women were. In this the National Woman's Party was well within the mainstream of medical opinion. Industrial physicians generally referred to women's wartime work favorably and discussed ways in which women workers differed little from male workers in capabilities. Also, evidence about lead's effects on the children of both male and female workers appeared in commonly used obstetrical and gynecological textbooks as early as 1917. The party's lack of criticism of fetal protection policies may be explained by the nature of the organization. Despite success in getting both major political party platforms to endorse the ERA beginning in 1944, by the 1950s, the National Woman's Party had become a small, one-issue organization largely comprising veterans from the ERA battles of the 1920s.[16]

Only Baetjer seems to have been poised to argue that while excessive exposure to lead prior to pregnancy might be dangerous to subsequent pregnancies, exposures that were "within safe limits, as defined for *adults* [emphasis added]," would present no hazard to women. Such arguments antedate those made in the 1970s, which called for safer workplaces for both men and women.[17]

Neither women nor men in the automobile industry protested fetal protection policies in the 1950s. In the next twenty-five years, however, the United Auto Workers (UAW), the Oil, Chemical and Atomic Workers Union, and the International Union of Electrical Workers confronted company fetal protection policies on behalf of their female and male members. The UAW filed the suit against Johnson Controls that resulted in the 1991 Supreme Court decision disallowing such policies.[18]

The immediate lack of response to fetal protection policies can perhaps be explained by examining the actions of women unionists in the 1950s. According to Nancy Gabin, these women "alternated between the poles of special protection and equal treatment." While women in heavily male occupations tended to believe that equal treatment offered the best opportunity for economic advancement, some women in the UAW believed that protective labor laws allowed working mothers time to take care of family responsibilities. Dorothy Sue Cobble has also pointed out that women in mostly female occupations like waiting on tables believed that sex typing could protect their jobs—even if the same women also supported the idea of equality. Many women, argues Cobble, sought to accommodate work to the reality of women's double duty. It is important to recognize the lingering existence of this ambivalence in the working class—male and female, unionized or not—about gender equality.[19]

Employment policies and legislation in the 1950s also demonstrate the tension between older and newer definitions of motherhood. Protective laws, which in the postwar era started to lose legitimacy, reified all the social tasks associated with motherhood and portrayed women as a group sharing similar social and cultural characteristics. Fetal protection policies around lead, while also based on the idea that women as a group shared characteristics, presumed that biology was *all* they shared. Moreover, fetal protection policies did seem to promise wider employment opportunities for women than were possible under traditional protective legislation governing hours. While a wide range of restrictions on overtime and night work could be justified on the grounds that women needed to be home to care properly for their families, policies crafted more narrowly around biology limited, at least theoretically, the number of prohibited jobs to those that posed significant biological risks to women's reproductive capacity. Nevertheless, fetal protection policies represented new methods of assigning group characteristics to women, reducing their rights to make individual choices and eventually reviving feminist perspectives on work and gender, particularly around equality and difference.

The American workplace had changed since the beginning of the century in other ways as well. Not only had it become more female, it had also become safer and healthier. Federal action in the 1930s had established minimum wage and maximum hours legislation across the country. State workers' compensation insurance provided an impetus for industry to reduce workplace hazards. Industrial advances in exhaust and ventilation engineering, changes in manufacturing and mining methods, scientific knowledge about chemicals and other materials, and medical discoveries in the treatment of disease had reduced dangers in the workplace to both men and women. This is not to say, however, that occupational illness in all industries decreased. In the late 1940s Hamilton described how the automobile manufacturing trade had become safer when painters began using lead-free lacquers, but then more dangerous after changes in body styles called for smoother lines, which were achieved by soldering seams with lead and then sanding them. The International Union of Mine, Mill and Smelter Workers told federal investigators in 1956 that the introduction of new mechanical devices in underground mines exposed workers to more silica, not less. Finally, in some industries, the extent of hazards caused by industrial materials with long latency periods, such as asbestos and ionizing radiation, was just beginning to surface.[20]

Growing interest in the number of environmental insults to the public and to workers prompted a number of studies on hazards specific to female workers. Following up on the 1958 detection of thesaurosis (a pulmonary disease resulting from the inhalation of hair spray), physicians in New York City in 1964 studied a group of beauticians (all female) against a control group (one-third female), and found no significant differences in lung capacity even among long-time hair spray users. (They did note differences between smokers and non-smokers.) They did not test women who used hair spray on their own hair, however, even though one physician had noted that "amateur home users" of toxic materials did not always know to take the measures necessary to protect themselves. In the case of beauticians, this was especially true, since they pointed the spray away from themselves in the shop, while home users directed the spray toward themselves.[21]

The growing percentage of women in the paid workforce—about one-third of all wage earners were women in 1960—also attracted medical attention. In 1961 the American Medical Association (AMA) prepared a new statement on women in industry, superseding the one it had issued in 1943. Developed by the AMA's Council on Occupational Health, the statement reflects many of the lessons of World War II, reducing the number of differences between men and women to essentially two: overall physical strength and pregnancy. The council acknowledged continued higher incidences of absenteeism among women but explained them in terms of women's dual responsibility toward work and toward home and family. The council also dismissed menstruation and menopause as significant causes of absenteeism because they could often be treated on the job with medication or with counseling. Pregnancy, however, merited detailed attention in nearly all aspects of work: the optimum number of working hours, the performance of certain tasks that might become logistically difficult in later months of pregnancy, and exposure to substances and processes known to be hazardous to fetuses, such as lead, benzene, and ionizing radiation.[22]

The significance of the AMA's document lies primarily in its specificity. Emphasizing the similar working conditions faced by men and women, the statement reflected many of the conditions detailed by Hamilton more than fifty years before, when she urged employers and physicians to restrict women from working at specific jobs and processes only if they were more dangerous to women than to men. The AMA's accent on unique biological characteristics rather than on social ones suggests a narrower definition of motherhood than the domesticity of the 1950s implies.

Even as the AMA came closer to recognizing the many roles women played and the varied physical characteristics they brought to the workplace, women workers began to recognize the selectivity with which many sex-specific employment rules, ostensibly aimed at protecting health, reinforced long-standing gender divisions of labor. Health activists in the women's movement began to write about the selectivity of excluded jobs, noting that ionizing radiation equipment routinely used by women in hospitals, for example, never seemed to appear on a list of jobs deemed too dangerous for women. On the other hand, higher paying jobs with the same risks were denied women for health reasons.[23]

Moreover, women familiar with the devastating impact of thalidomide on children born to women who had trustingly used the drug in the early 1960s while pregnant did not automatically depend on industry's pronouncements on the health and safety of a product or a process based on scientific evidence. They began to prefer their own research. One result was the 1971 publication of the pathbreaking *Our Bodies, Ourselves* by the Boston Women's Health Book Collective.[24]

Health activists also criticized what they viewed as inadequate medical evidence and experience, again based on gender assumptions. For instance, scientists almost always studied reproductive hazards in women workers, despite growing evidence about and concern by male workers that healthy fatherhood might be at risk. Conversely, employers often used male standards of physical strength or susceptibility to temperature, for example, as employment norms for all workers, regardless of whether those characteristics were actually necessary in order to perform the particular job. Women who did not meet the standards believed themselves to be unfairly excluded from these positions. For many, male-defined notions of behavior became the standard against which women felt compelled to judge themselves.[25]

Employment norms, which seemed to move into public consciousness in the 1960s and which set the stage for debates over gender and employment in the 1970s, had actually been in flux since World War II. Employers who had commonly imposed sex-based pay differentials found themselves stymied by changes in employment and placement determinations during the war. Once employers or managers had to begin looking at individual rather than gender differences among workers, it became difficult to consider women as a homogeneous group—although many continued to try. After the war, women workers who had wanted employment in higher paying blue-collar jobs made numerous efforts to reorganize job descriptions based on the specific attributes required rather than on traditional sex-based categories. But it was an uphill battle. Not surprisingly, once such changes did begin to occur, male unionists often supported women's efforts for equitable pay structures: men did not want to see their jobs filled by women at lower pay.[26]

Women's advancement in the workplace became somewhat easier in the 1960s. The influence of the civil-rights movement and the eventual passage of the 1964 Civil Rights Act, which outlawed sex and race discrimination in employment, improved women's legal rights, at least, to equal employment.[27]

Despite the passage of the Civil Rights Act, however, state protective legislation tended to remain on the books, causing a great deal of confusion for employers. Sex-discrimination charges brought by women workers who appealed to the newly created Equal Employment Opportunity Commission (EEOC) often ran counter to the letter of the now outdated statutes. In many cases commissioners recommended that employers apply to their respective state labor board for exceptions to sex-based protective laws. In Pennsylvania these cases resulted in amendments to the laws. In 1966 Marjorie Stanchak was denied a promotion to the position of draw furnace operator at the Screw and Bolt Corporation of America in Pittsburgh because it was described as a seven-day-a-week, eight-hour-a-day job with no scheduled rest breaks. This violated laws requiring employers to grant women a thirty-minute break after five hours of work and a forty-eight-hour maximum weekly limit. As a result of such situations, the state legislature eliminated maximum hours for women as unenforceable, especially if women had more than one job, and allowed companies to make written application for exemptions to the rules regarding rest periods. For the EEOC, however, problems remained, since it was unclear whether the state would allow for the complete elimination of a rest break, or require employers to institute two shorter breaks. Moreover, under Pennsylvania law, women workers themselves had the option of waiving the rest requirement. The variety of work rules and state legislation created a number of conundrums for the EEOC in the late 1960s. By 1970, however, nearly all sex-based state labor legislation had been either eliminated or expanded to include male workers.[28]

Pregnancy-related discrimination cases had begun to wind their way through the courts by this time, and they posed different employment questions. Lise Vogel has described strategies for challenging pregnancy-related employment discrimination from two perspectives, one rooted in gender equality and one rooted in gender difference. As in the 1920s, feminists in the 1970s again divided over the means of achieving "equality."[29]

In the late 1960s one group of feminists argued strongly that pregnancy was only one condition of many similar ones that temporarily disabled men and women workers. Pregnancy leave, therefore, should be treated as a temporary disability comparable to other temporary conditions experienced by male and female workers. Another group viewed pregnancy as a condition particular to some women; a leave policy that dealt only with the limited physical needs associated with pregnancy provided "real equality" because it recognized women's unique biological difference from men. While seeking to limit "difference" to biology, these feminists argued that women as mothers deserved special consideration for their child-rearing abilities and should not be forced to fit into male-defined models of workplace behavior.[30]

In their belief that separating child-rearing from childbearing might provide women workers with the theoretical framework they needed to challenge sex discrimination arising from motherhood, both groups of feminists finally linked up with a position that had been evolving since the second decade of the twentieth century. The resulting Pregnancy Discrimination Act, passed in 1978, did not resolve feminist differences, but it did provide the framework both parties sought.[31]

The enactment of a federal Occupational Safety and Health Act in 1970, as well as the foundation of a research institute—the National Institute on Occupational Safety and Health (NIOSH)—enhanced the efforts of labor and women's activists concerned with working conditions. In 1975 the prestigious American Academy for the Advancement of Science sponsored a symposium on the occupational health status of women. Like reformers at the turn of the century, participants in the conference believed that women were not sufficiently safe in the workplace, and speakers particularly targeted various maternal issues. This conference, however, centered around both the specific biological hazards in the workplace and the health implications of paying attention to such hazards. While applauding the achievements of the women's movement, Vilma Hunt wondered if it had inadvertently caused an absence of scientific research and literature on health hazards specific to working women. She worried that the paucity of good research might lead to unjustified and extreme protective measures aimed at women or, just as unfortunate in her mind, inadequate consideration of sex-specific characteristics when criteria were being set. Hunt listed fetal protection policies as one example, not dismissing them as inherently discriminatory. Instead, she suggested that such policies required intense scrutiny.[32]

Andrea Hricko agreed. She believed that the women's rights movement in the 1960s and 1970s had actually hindered scientific research into the problems of pregnant women. She reported, however, that some of the sex-specific research that was being done had yielded some surprising results: one NIOSH study found an increased risk of birth defects not only in the offspring of female operating room personnel but also in the children born to unexposed wives of male operating room workers.[33]

Other speakers rejected the notion that excluding women workers from a particular workplace environment meant that the workplace was safe for all workers. David Wegman used data on reproductive hazards to women to argue for "more extensive medical and engineering control measures, not exclusion." Men, he went on, also needed adequate workplace controls.[34]

Jeanne Mager Stellman, a toxicologist with the American Health Foundation, strongly agreed. Fetal protection policies are discriminatory, she stated, because they assume that "just because a woman *can* bear children, it is presumed that she *will* bear children—the perpetual pregnancy myth [emphasis in original]." Moreover, she described efforts at excluding women from the "leaded" workplace while ignoring lead's effects on men as neither "safeguard[ing] human reproduction nor prevent[ing] the children already born from suffering the effects of lead."[35]

In spite of these protests, however, by the mid- to late 1970s at least fifteen Fortune 500 companies and numerous hospitals had introduced policies that in some way excluded fertile or pregnant women from some jobs deemed dangerous to the fetus. Exxon's medical director, Norbert Roberts, clearly stated the economic position of business when he announced publicly, "Our recommendation probably will be that women of child-bearing age should not be exposed to benzene until the facts are in. If we don't take such action, we may be in trouble scientifically; and if we do, we may be in trouble legally. But we'd rather face the EEOC than a deformed baby."[36]

According to the Congressional Office of Technology Assessment (OTA), corporate policies ranged from formal and epidemiologically based to anecdotal and informal, but all purported to be "scientifically justified," a claim the OTA sometimes questioned. DuPont listed seven substances from which "females of childbearing capability" would be excluded. Shell categorized dangerous jobs in terms of fetotoxicity or teratogenicity (poisonous only to the fetus or causing genetic damage, respectively).[37]

The best-known case during this period involved American Cyanamid's fetal protection policy, initiated in January 1978. Its most controversial aspect was the surgical sterilization of five women—allegedly with the encouragement of the industrial relations department and the plant medical staff. In early 1980 women who had transferred out of excluded areas or had been sterilized to keep jobs considered off-limits by the fetal protection policies, sued American Cyanamid under the 1964 Civil Rights Act. The company settled before going to trial but admitted no liability. The OTA believed that the company's policy had been initiated "with little scientific justification and little sensitivity to the needs of the workers," although the company's medical director strongly disagreed.[38]

One observer in 1980 correctly predicted that fetal protection policies would become the major occupational health issue of the 1980s, and indeed, legal challenges increased during that period. Some women workers (and the unions) challenged these policies through arbitration. Sally Kenney has argued that the passage of the Pregnancy Discrimination Act in 1978 provided a base from which to challenge them on constitutional grounds. Such efforts eventually resulted in the 1991 Supreme Court decision in *UAW v. Johnson Controls, Inc.*, which called such policies unconstitutional under the Pregnancy Discrimination Act of the 1964 Civil Rights Act.[39]

The apparent magnitude of changes in the workplace in the thirty years covered by this chapter is in many ways just that—apparent. Many of the workplace health policies of the 1980s had been in place since 1950, especially those that favored scientific research on highly targeted aspects of disease. Gender norms, in contrast, seem to have changed a great deal, although they, too, derived from attitudes that could be seen in 1950. In assessing the effects of and the attention paid to both, it is important first to consider the presumed benefits derived from science and feminism, and then to consider their influence on each other.

Reliance on medicine's ability to pinpoint specific pathogens as disease-causing agents led to the identification and control of many workplace hazards. But as David Rosner, Gerald Markowitz, and others have pointed out, practitioners of modern science tended both to reject the notion that a dangerous material could be eliminated from the workplace and to ignore the interaction of a number of environmental factors in the workplace that adversely affected health.

Ideas about gender also affected the workplace health of male and female workers. Historically, movements to promote gender equality in the workplace resulted in the increased use of individual standards of employment, some of which served to increase employer scrutiny of the private lives of workers. Such policies, however, could also protect some male workers from jobs that were beyond their physical strength. Similarly, special treatment for women workers in many cases led to changes in working conditions that improved the lives of all workers. But policies that treated women differently also tended to skew medical research toward female reproductive dangers—to the exclusion of similar research on men.

Because gender roles changed so visibly between 1950 and 1980, it is tempting to argue that gender exerted more influence on occupational health policies than did medical science. In fact, the advent of federal legislation around health and the environment sparked numerous studies on reproductive health hazards to both men and women. This interaction between medicine and gender has continued to prompt a variety of approaches to workplace health. It is important to recognize the trade-offs associated with emphasizing one explanation over another; it is also important to keep asking the questions.

Epilogue

One of the more significant lessons behind efforts to eliminate sex discrimination in the workplace must be that each strategy is situated in a particular context. In the international arena, for instance, Chinese activists seek to emphasize a woman's uniqueness, her motherhood, while the Namibian constitution authorizes affirmative action for women and forbids sex discrimination. In countless nations women have drawn on their power as mothers to forge a political identity. For example, in the 1970s Argentina's Mothers of the Plaza de Mayo formed in order to demand accountability from an authoritarian government. In the United States, Filipino women have used the gender stereotypes espoused by their male supervisors to gain short-term improvements in working conditions. Sometimes medical research can be used in the same way. While the discovery of premenstrual syndrome in the 1980s was used by some as a justification for discriminatory practices, some women workers used this evidence to acknowledge bona fide illness.[1]

In attempting transnational alliances among women's groups organizing around workplace health, we need to bear in mind the costs of each strategy. Understanding historical roots and political, cultural, medical, and economic consequences may offer possibilities for improving workplace conditions for men and women in developing nations. As in the United States earlier in the twentieth century, women's organizations in India have been conducting surveys of employed women, filling a gap left by organized labor. An organization in the Dominican Republic has been researching the health and working conditions of industrial homework.[2]

Progress has been made, I believe, in recognizing how the particular circumstances of women's lives have influenced workplace environments for both men and women. Recognition that some women are mothers has resulted in nursing rooms in the Pentagon as well as a Family and Medical Leave Act available to mothers and fathers. The re-engineering of equipment to reduce lifting loads for women not only reduced back injuries for men as well, but also led to ergonomic changes in the workplace for men and women.

But we need to be careful in applauding the effects of feminizing the workplace. A recent study in this country indicated that women, especially mothers, are more stressed at work than men. For wage-earning mothers, this study must have seemed like a waste of research money. Now, as before, the double day of mothers who work outside the home is recognized as a health issue that affects productivity in the workplace. And now, as before, this evidence could be used to change the workplace environment—or it could become a rationale for excluding women from the workplace. While it is appropriate to recognize that a person's health should be viewed in a much broader context than the rather narrow environment of the workplace, we continue to run the risk of allowing employers to avoid responsibility for conditions in their plants that might be sources of illness.

Remember *Johnson Controls*. Feminists who opposed fetal protection policies promoted environmental changes in the workplace and demanded that employers allow women workers, like their male counterparts, to make their own decisions about parenthood. The feminist "victory" over Johnson Controls in the Supreme Court must be tempered by the realization that the decision did not result in a different work environment. Emphasizing equal rights has placed responsibility for health on the workers themselves. As in the earlier period, without changes in the environment, remedies for occupational safety and health hazards have tended to focus on very specific regulation of materials, machines, and individual behavior.[3] Ideas about gender equality and difference carry consequences that both advance and retard women's status in the workplace.

The economics of doing business drives management decisions. Johnson Controls' reasons for implementing fetal protection policies were rooted in the financial uncertainty raised by the specter of a lawsuit—a child suing the company for harm done, in utero, while his or her mother worked at the plant. This issue was not resolved by the Supreme Court. We need better ways of responding to employers who determine they must balance their economic imperatives against the state's insistence on equal treatment. How companies are treated may play a significant role in determining whether they choose to maintain operations in this country or move elsewhere. In either case, improving occupational health and safety conditions must be seen in a global context.[4]

Finally, attitudes about motherhood continue to inform our lives. It is necessary to look more closely at how modern science has served as a double-edged sword for women. Its specific attention to physiology offered a means by which gender roles could be separated from biological capabilities, theoretically widening women's work opportunities and excluding women from only those jobs that adversely affected their ability to bear healthy children. Conversely, medical evidence about poisons with an emphasis on reproduction also gave new authority to those who wanted to use biology to emphasize women's differences from men. Discerning the relative importance of science in shaping the attention we pay to gender in the workplace may offer clues to broader social issues.[5]

Advances in reproductive technology, coupled with increasingly strident calls for fetal rights, complicate the understanding of motherhood, in many cases sending mixed messages. Young women who are potential (or actual) egg donors for infertile women are encouraged to de-emphasize the biological aspects of mothering; the egg recipient defines motherhood by her ability to carry this embryo to term. Societal responses to women's prenatal activities also reflect conflicting values. While the Supreme Court grants a woman autonomy over her own body with respect to abortion, some laws also seek to criminalize a pregnant woman who drinks too much or uses drugs, both of which can put her fetus at risk.[6]

As in the past, we must continue to look beyond the tendency for science and technology to define and delimit this aspect of *some* women's lives as the determining factor in *all* women's lives. But we also need to be aware of how assumptions about motherhood permeate culture in this country and around the world, placing motherhood squarely within the political and economic mainstream. It is possible to appreciate the long-lasting nature of contemporary concerns—and also the potential for change. By examining how these ideas translate into policy, organizations focused on women's health and human rights can create strategies for improving the status of women around the world.

Abbreviations

AHP-SL	Alice Hamilton Papers. Schlesinger Library, Radcliffe College, Harvard University Libraries. Cambridge, Massachusetts.
ALP-SL	Alma Lutz Papers. Schlesinger Library, Radcliffe College, Harvard University Libraries. Cambridge, Massachusetts.
AMWA-MCP	American Medical Women's Association. Medical College of Pennsylvania Archives and Special Collections on Women in Medicine. Philadelphia.
BCC-BL	Boston Chamber of Commerce Papers. Baker Library Manuscripts and Special Collections, Harvard University Libraries. Cambridge, Massachusetts.
CLC-SL	Consumers' League of Connecticut Papers. Schlesinger Library, Radcliffe College, Harvard University Libraries. Cambridge, Massachusetts.
CLM-SL	Consumers' League of Massachusetts Papers. Schlesinger Library, Radcliffe College, Harvard University Libraries. Cambridge, Massachusetts.
CLNJ-RU	Consumers' League of New Jersey Papers. Special Collections and Archives, Rutgers University Libraries. New Brunswick, New Jersey.
DIH-NYS	New York State Division of Industrial Hygiene Medical Reference Files, 1929–1973. New York State Department of Labor, New York State Archives. Albany.
EC-SSC	Smith College Employment Collection. Sophia Smith Collection, Smith College. Northampton, Massachusetts.
EFW-SSC	Emma France Ward Papers. Sophia Smith Collection, Smith College. Northampton, Massachusetts.
HLH-SL	Harriet L. Hardy Papers. Schlesinger Library, Radcliffe College, Harvard University Libraries. Cambridge, Massachusetts.

KBS-MCP	Katharine Boucot Sturgis Papers. Medical College of Pennsylvania Archives and Special Collections on Women in Medicine. Philadelphia.
MGH-SSD	Massachusetts General Hospital Social Service Department Records. Massachusetts General Hospital. Boston.
MRA-BL	Manufacturers' Research Association Papers. Baker Library Manuscripts and Special Collections, Harvard University Libraries. Cambridge, Massachusetts.
MvK-SSC	Mary van Kleeck Papers. Sophia Smith Collection, Smith College. Northampton, Massachusetts.
MWIA-MCP	Medical Women's International Association Papers. Medical College of Pennsylvania Archives and Special Collections on Women in Medicine. Philadelphia.
NCL-LC	National Consumers' League Papers. Library of Congress. Washington, D.C.
RBF-RAC	Rockefeller Brothers Fund Papers. Rockefeller Archives Center. Tarrytown, New York.
SA-UML	Survey Associates Papers. Social Welfare History Archives, University of Minnesota Libraries. Minneapolis.
WB-NA	Women's Bureau of the U.S. Department of Labor Records. National Archives and Records Administration. College Park, Maryland.

Notes

Introduction

1. Linda Gordon's "maternalism" is spelled out in her *Pitied but Not Entitled: Single Mothers and the History of Welfare, 1890–1935.*

2. For a discussion of science and womanhood at the turn of the century, see Cynthia Eagle Russett, *Sexual Science: The Victorian Construction of Womanhood;* Barbara Sicherman, "Working It Out: Gender, Profession and Reform in the Career of Alice Hamilton," in *Gender, Class, Race, and Reform in the Progressive Era,* ed. Noralee Frankel and Nancy Schrom Dye; Rima Apple, ed., *Women, Health, and Medicine: A Historical Handbook;* and Richard A. Meckel, *Save the Babies: American Public Health Reform and the Prevention of Infant Mortality, 1850–1929.* For analyses of more recent events, especially fetal protection policies, see Sally Kenney, *For Whose Protection? Reproductive Hazards and Exclusionary Policies in the United States and Great Britain;* Robert Blank, *Fetal Protection in the Workplace: Women's Rights, Business Interests, and the Unborn;* and Cynthia R. Daniels, *At Women's Expense: State Power and the Politics of Fetal Rights.*

3. For accounts of the rise of scientific medicine, see Charles E. Rosenberg, "The Therapeutic Revolution: Medicine, Meaning, and Social Change in Nineteenth-Century America," 3–25; and Stanley Joel Reiser, *Medicine and the Reign of Technology.* Many historians have examined the impact of medical authority on women's lives, including Carroll Smith-Rosenberg, *Disorderly Conduct: Visions of Gender in Victorian America;* Judith Walzer Leavitt, *Brought to Bed: Childbirth in America, 1750–1950* (Oxford: Oxford University Press, 1986); James Reed, *The Birth Control Movement and American Society: From Private Vice to Public Virtue;* and Linda Gordon, *Woman's Body, Woman's Right: A Social History of Birth Control in America.* Judith Walzer Leavitt's *Healthiest City: Milwaukee and the Politics of Health Reform* provides a good survey of the overlap between "old" and "new" medicine in the realm of public health, as does Charles E. Rosenberg's *No Other Gods: On Science and American Social Thought.*

4. Samuel P. Hays and Barbara D. Hays, *Beauty, Health, and Permanence: Environmental Politics in the United States, 1955–1985;* Donald Worster, *The Wealth of Nature: Environmental History and the Ecological Imagination;* and Richard Smith, "Environmental History, Ecology and Meaning," *Journal of American History* 76 (March 1990). See also "A Round Table: Environmental History," *Journal of American History* 76 (March 1990).

5. Carolyn Merchant, *Ecological Revolutions: Nature, Gender, and Science in New England; Women and Environmental History,* special issue of *Environmental Review.*

6. Nicholas Freudenberg and Ellen Zaltzberg, "From Grassroots Activism to Political Power: Women Organizing against Environmental Hazards," in Chavkin, ed., *Double Exposure,* 246–72. Christopher C. Sellers, in *Hazards of the Job: From Industrial Disease to Environmental Health Science,* argues that postwar environmentalism has its roots in industrial hygiene activity in the early part of this century, although he does not examine how gender influenced both of these movements.

7. Few historians of protective legislation have considered the medical and scientific rationales for sex-specific laws. Alice Kessler-Harris, *Out to Work: A History of Wage-Earning Women in the United States;* Ann Corinne Hill, "Protection of Women Workers and the Courts: A Legal Case History"; Vilma Hunt, "A Brief History of Women Workers and Hazards in the Workplace"; Rosalind Petchesky, "Workers, Reproductive Hazards and the Politics of Protection: An Introduction"; Judith Scott, "Keeping Women in Their Place: Exclusionary Policies and Reproduction"; Patricia Vawter Klein, "'For the Good of the Race': Reproductive Hazards from Lead and the Persistence of Exclusionary Policies toward Women"; Susan Lehrer, *Origins of Protective Labor Legislation for Women, 1905–1925.*

8. For labor's perspective on the sex-segregated workplace, see Nancy Gabin, *Feminism in the Labor Movement: Women and the United Auto Workers, 1935–1975,* and Kessler-Harris, *Out to Work.* Lise Vogel, *Mothers on the Job: Maternity Policy in the United States,* has studied the policy implications of difference in the workplace. The politics of difference is described in various publications, for example, Ruth Milkman, "Women's History and the Sears Case"; Kenney, *For Whose Protection?* and Joan R. Scott, "Gender as a Useful Category of Analysis." For accounts of the history of modern feminism, see Nancy F. Cott, *The Grounding of Modern Feminism;* Leila Rupp and Verta Taylor, *Survival in the Doldrums: The American Women's Rights Movement, 1945 to the 1960s;* Robyn Muncy, *Creating a Female Dominion in American Reform;* Wendy Sarvasy, "Beyond the Difference versus Equality Debate: Postsuffrage Feminism, Citizenship, and the Quest for the Feminist Welfare State"; and Kathryn Kish Sklar, "Why Were Most Politically Active Women Opposed to the ERA in the 1920s?"

9. Barbara Sicherman, *Alice Hamilton: A Life in Letters;* Rupp and Taylor, *Survival in the Doldrums.*

10. *International Union, United Automobile Workers v. Johnson Controls, Inc.,* 111 S.Ct. 1196 (1991).

Chapter 1

1. Robert Watchorn, *Fifth Annual Report of the Factory Inspectors* (Harrisburg: Commonwealth of Pennsylvania, 1894), 455.

2. Watchorn, *Fifth Annual Report,* 456. Shoddy mills manufactured yarn, fabric, or garments from shredded woolen rags or worn clothing.

3. David Rosner and Gerald Markowitz, *Deadly Dust: Silicosis and the Politics of Occupational Disease in Twentieth-Century America,* 218–9.

4. Robert H. Wiebe, *The Search for Order, 1877–1920.*

5. Charles E. Rosenberg, "The Therapeutic Revolution: Medicine, Meaning, and Social Change in Nineteenth-Century America."

6. See, for example, John Duffy, *A History of Public Health in New York City;* Stuart Galishoff, *Safeguarding the Public Health: Newark, 1895–1918;* Judith Walzer Leavitt, *The Healthiest City: Milwaukee and the Politics of Health Reform;* Charles E. Rosenberg, *The Cholera Years: The United States in 1832, 1849, and 1866;* and Barbara Gutmann Rosenkrantz, *Public Health and the State: Changing Views in Massachusetts, 1842–1936.*

7. Exhibit in Boott Cotton Mills Museum, Lowell National Historic Park, Lowell, Massachusetts.

8. Elizabeth Stuart Phelps, *The Silent Partner,* 81, 119, 232.

9. Alice Kessler-Harris, *Out to Work: A History of Wage-Earning Women in the United States,* 184. See also Patricia Reeve, "Injured in the Service of the Commonwealth: Massachusetts Industrial Soldiers Seek Recompense, 1881–1887."

10. Eileen Boris, *Home to Work: Motherhood and the Politics of Industrial Homework in the United States,* 171–98.

11. Watchorn, *Fifth Annual Report,* 39, 45.

12. *State of New Jersey Reports* (Trenton: Department of Labor, 1906, 1907, 1908).

13. Quoted in David Rosner and Gerald Markowitz, "The Early Movement for Occupational Safety and Health, 1900–1917," 511.

14. James Campbell, *Eighth Annual Report of the Factory Inspectors* (Harrisburg: Commonwealth of Pennsylvania, 1897), 650.

15. Mary Putnam Jacobi, *Report and Testimony Taken before the Special (Reinhard) Committee of the Assembly Appointed to Investigate the Condition of Female Labor in the City of New York,* January 16, 1896, cited in Josephine Goldmark, *Fatigue and Efficiency: A Study in Industry,* 507.

16. Agnes deLima, "Night-Working Mothers in Textile Mills, Passaic, New Jersey" (Consumers' League of New Jersey, December 1920), p. 13, folder "Industrial Relations, Pamphlets," EC-SSC.

17. Ibid., p. 12.

18. *New York State Department of Labor Bulletin,* no. 8: *1906* (1907), 11, 12, 36, 39, cited in "Organizational and Planning Files Concerning Advisory Committees on the Proposed Labor Law Recodification," records of the New York State Factory Investigating Commission, New York State Archives and Records Administration, Albany.

19. Carl Gersuny, *Work Hazards and Industrial Conflict,* 41, 44.

20. Annie Nathan Meyer, *Women's Work in America* (New York: Henry Holt, 1891), 310–1.

21. Cynthia Eagle Russett, *Sexual Science: The Victorian Construction of Womanhood,* 156, 158; *Report of the Nebraska Bureau of Labor and Industrial Studies, 1907–1908,* 33, cited in Goldmark, *Fatigue and Efficiency,* 251; *Report of the Michigan Bureau of Labor, 1908,* 337, cited in Goldmark, *Fatigue and Efficiency,* 268.

22. Russett, *Sexual Science*, 172; Charles E. Rosenberg, *No Other Gods: On Science and American Social Thought*, 25–53. See also Carl Degler, *In Search of Human Nature: The Decline and Revival of Darwinism in American Social Thought*.

23. Poster, "How to Avoid Common Colds," and "Report on Common Colds by the Committee on Prevention of Disease, December 1910," case 64, BCC-BL.

24. Carter's Ink Company to James Honeij, November 22, 1910, case 64, BCC-BL.

25. "Summary of Conclusions, January 10, 1911," case 64, BCC-BL.

26. Publications and letters, organized by region, folder 332–19, "Industrial Welfare Work—Pennsylvania and New Jersey, 1913," box 48, BCC-BL.

27. "The Home of the 57" (H.J. Heinz Company, n.d.), folder 332–19, "Industrial Welfare Work—Pennsylvania and New Jersey, 1913," pp. 26–8, 33, box 48, BCC-BL.

28. Brighton Mills to James Honeij, April 19, 1913, folder 332–19, "Industrial Welfare Work—Pennsylvania and New Jersey, 1913," box 48, BCC-BL; E. J. Barcalo to James McKibben, May 1, 1913, folder 332–19, "Industrial Welfare Work—New York, 1913," box 48, BCC-BL; report from Marshall Field and Company, April 19, 1913, folder 332–19, "Industrial Welfare Work in Ohio, Wisconsin, Missouri, Louisiana, Illinois, Michigan, 1910–1913," box 48, BCC-BL. See also Jill E. Cooper, "Keeping the Girls on the Line: The Medical Department and Women Workers at AT&T, 1913–1940," paper presented at the annual meeting of the American Association for the History of Medicine, Buffalo, New York, May 12, 1996.

29. Wade Wright, "Physical Exams" (Metropolitan Life Insurance Company, n.d.), folder 332–19, "Industrial Welfare Work, Misc., 1910–1925," box 48, BCC-BL.

30. Charles H. Hulburd to Boston Chamber of Commerce, April 8, 1913, folder 332–19, "Industrial Welfare Work in Ohio, Wisconsin, Missouri, Louisiana, Illinois, Michigan, 1910–1913," box 48, BCC-BL; E. Seward to Boston Chamber of Commerce, May 10, 1913, folder 332–19, "Industrial Relations Welfare Work—New England, 1913," box 48, BCC-BL.

31. E. L. Nazro, "Industrial Relations, June 11, 1909," folder 332–19, "Industrial Relations Welfare Work, Profit-Sharing, Cleveland, Ohio, Boston, and Misc., 1909–1917," box 48, BCC-BL.

32. See, for example, Susan Porter Benson's *Counter Cultures: Saleswomen, Managers and Customers in American Department Stores, 1890–1940*. See also Reeve, "Injured in the Service of the Commonwealth"; and Alan Derickson, "Physiological Science and Scientific Management in the Progressive Era: Frederic S. Lee and the Committee on Industrial Fatigue."

33. See, for example, folder 332–19, box 48, BCC-BL; and folder, "Miscellaneous Court Cases," box CR-5, Amoskeag Manufacturing Company Papers, Baker Library Manuscripts Collection, Harvard University. See also Christopher Sellers, "Public Health Service's Office of Industrial Hygiene and the Transformation of Industrial Medicine."

34. E. J. Barcalo to James McKibben, May 1, 1913, folder 332–19, "Industrial Welfare Work—New York, 1913," box 48, BCC-BL.

Notes to Chapter 1

35. Wiebe, *Search for Order,* 111–32.
36. Ibid.
37. Ibid., 168–70, 154.
38. Rosenberg, "Therapeutic Revolution," 3–25; Rosemary Stevens, *American Medicine and the Public Interest.*
39. Leavitt, *Healthiest City,* 243–6; John Duffy, "Social Impact of Disease in the Late Nineteenth Century," 420.
40. Morris J. Vogel, *The Invention of the Modern Hospital: Boston, 1870–1930,* 27; Ida M. Cannon, *On the Social Frontier of Medicine: Pioneering in Medical Social Service,* 179; Jean Alonzo Curran, *Founders: Harvard School of Public Health,* 182.
41. Richard Cabot, *First Annual Report of Social Work Permitted at the Massachusetts General Hospital, October 1, 1905 to October 1, 1906,* p. 9, MGH-SSD; Richard Cabot, *Third Annual Report of the Social Service Department of the Massachusetts General Hospital, October 1, 1907 to October 1, 1908,* p. 10, MGH-SSD; Neva Deardorff, "Cabot, Richard Clarke," in *Dictionary of American Biography,* vol. 22, suppl. 2, 84.
42. Cannon had started her career at Massachusetts General as a volunteer but soon began working with Cabot to compensate for the shortcomings in institutional care. Cannon, *On the Social Frontier of Medicine,* 181; Morris J. Vogel, "Cannon, Ida Maud," in *Dictionary of American Biography,* suppl. 6, 97–8.
43. Richard Cabot, *First Annual Report,* p. 20, MGH-SSD.
44. Roger I. Lee, *Sixth Annual Report of the Social Service Department of the Massachusetts General Hospital, January 1, 1911 to January 1, 1912,* pp. 20–21, MGH-SSD.
45. Curran, *Founders: Harvard School of Public Health,* 184; Mary Van Kleeck, "Memorandum Regarding Occupational Investigations at Massachusetts General Hospital, September 24, 1914," p. 5, folder 132, Department of Industrial Studies, Series IV4B1, Russell Sage Foundation Papers, Rockefeller Archives Center, Tarrytown, New York.
46. *State of New Jersey Report* (Trenton: Department of Labor, 1911), 12; Rosner and Markowitz, "Early Movement," 512.
47. Kessler-Harris, *Out to Work,* 186; *Commonwealth v. Beatty,* 15 Pa. Superior Court 5 (1900), 8.
48. Nancy Woloch, *Muller v. Oregon: A Brief History with Documents,* 28–9; Louis D. Brandeis, Brief for the Defendant, Supreme Court of the United States, October Term 1907, *Curt Muller v. State of Oregon,* 24, 28, 36; Louis D. Brandeis and Josephine Goldmark, *Women in Industry: Decision of the United States Supreme Court in Curt Muller vs. State of Oregon* (reprint, National Consumers' League, New York, 1908), 6.
49. *Commonwealth of Pennsylvania Legislative Journal* 1 (1913): 1180–6; Alice Hamilton, "Possibilities and Limitations of the Employment of Women in Industry," *Monthly Bulletin of the Pennsylvania Department of Labor and Industry* 5 (1918): 37; Susan Lehrer, *Origins of Protective Labor Legislation for Women, 1905–1925,* 126–40. See also Ann Corinne Hill, "Protection of Women Workers and the Courts: A Legal Case History."

50. "Working Hours for Women," *American Association for Labor Legislation Review* 6 (December 1916): 372–81.

51. Christopher Sellers, "Office of Industrial Hygiene," 45–9, has noted a similar trend.

52. Josephine Goldmark, *Fatigue and Efficiency*; Robert Bremner, "Goldmark, Josephine Clara," in *Notable American Women, 1607–1950*, 2:60.

53. See, for example, Regina Markell Morantz-Sanchez, *Sympathy and Science: Women Physicians in American Medicine;* and James Harvey Young, "Patent Medicines and the Self-Help Syndrome." For an updated analysis of fatigue, see Edward Shorter, *From Paralysis to Fatigue: A History of Psychosomatic Illness in the Modern Era.*

54. Goldmark, *Fatigue and Efficiency*, 90, 95.

55. Ibid. See also Derickson, "Physiological Science."

56. Frederick Winslow Taylor, quoted in Derickson, "Physiological Science," 501, 502.

57. Alfred Barlow, *The History and Principles of Weaving by Hand and by Power,* 268 (with thanks to Maryrose Lane, Park Ranger at the Lowell National Historical Park, National Park Service, Lowell, Massachusetts, for this citation).

58. Phelps, *The Silent Partner;* William Mass and Charles Levenstein, "Labor Relations, Technology, and Occupational Disease: Banning the Suck Shuttle in Massachusetts, 1911," 7, 19–26 (with thanks to Patricia Reeve for the citation); Gersuny, *Work Hazards and Industrial Conflict,* 7.

59. Allen F. Davis, *American Heroine: The Life and Legend of Jane Addams.*

60. Leavitt, *Healthiest City.*

Chapter 2

1. Alice Hamilton, "Possibilities and Limitations of the Employment of Women in Industry," *Monthly Bulletin of the Pennsylvania Department of Labor and Industry* 5 (1918): 37, 39.

2. Carroll Smith-Rosenberg, *Disorderly Conduct: Visions of Gender in Victorian America,* 237, 236; James Reed, *The Birth Control Movement and American Society: From Private Vice to Public Virtue,* x, 45; Linda Gordon, *Woman's Body, Woman's Right: A Social History of Birth Control in America,* 254, 95–7.

3. Cynthia Eagle Russett, *Sexual Science: The Victorian Construction of Womanhood,* 120, 112, 123, 206. See also Reed, *Birth Control Movement,* 40–3. The scientific basis of racism is described by Stephen Jay Gould in *The Mismeasure of Man.*

4. Judith Walzer Leavitt, *Brought to Bed: Childbirth in America, 1750–1950* (Oxford: Oxford University Press, 1986), 102–6.

5. Margaret Marsh and Wanda Ronner, *The Empty Cradle: Infertility in America from Colonial Times to the Present,* 84.

6. Marsh and Ronner, *Empty Cradle,* 83. See also Allen F. Davis, *American Heroine: The Life and Legend of Jane Addams;* Judith Walzer Leavitt, *The Healthiest City: Milwaukee and the Politics of Health Reform,* 194–200; Richard A. Meckel, *Save the Babies:*

American Public Health Reform and the Prevention of Infant Mortality, 1850–1929; and Allen F. Davis, *Spearheads for Reform: The Social Settlements and the Progressive Movement, 1890–1914.*

7. Ida M. Cannon, *Third Annual Report of the Social Service Department of the Massachusetts General Hospital, October 1, 1907 to October 1, 1908,* p. 37, MGH-SSD. See also Julie Berebitsky, "'Like' Our Very Own: Adoptive Parenthood in the United States, 1870–1945."

8. Reed, *Birth Control Movement,* 225–77. See also Meckel, *Save the Babies.*

9. Protective labor legislation has received substantial scholarly attention, particularly with respect to its impact on equal rights legislation for women and on women's advancement in nontraditional occupations. Historians of women have usually placed the issue of industrial reproductive hazards completely within the feminist debate over hours limitations and have failed to consider it as a separate issue—or else have ignored it. If the subject of poisons appears at all, it usually does so under the "working conditions" part of "hours and working conditions." See Nancy F. Cott, *The Grounding of Modern Feminism;* Alice Kessler-Harris, *Out to Work: A History of Wage-Earning Women in the United States;* Claudia Goldin, *Understanding the Gender Gap: An Economic History of American Women;* and Susan Lehrer, *Origins of Protective Labor Legislation for Women, 1905–1925.*

Scholars who focus on present-day concerns about occupational threats to women's reproductive systems have asserted the historical existence of these concerns but have not analyzed their failure or success in policy and legislative arenas. See, for example, Carolyn Bell, "Implementing Safety and Health Regulations for Women in the Workplace"; Ann Corinne Hill, "Protection of Workers in the Workplace: Implications for the Equal Rights of Women," *Feminist Studies* 5 (Summer 1979): 247–73; Michael Wright, "Reproductive Hazards and 'Protective' Discrimination"; Wendy Chavkin, ed., *Double Exposure: Women's Health Hazards on the Job and at Home;* and Ruth Heifetz, "Women, Lead, and Reproductive Hazards: Defining a New Risk."

Historians of occupational health and safety have expanded our knowledge about the origins, directions, and scientific, political, and economic implications of occupational disease, but they have only recently begun to explore how gender intersected these points. See David Rosner and Gerald Markowitz, "The Early Movement for Occupational Safety and Health, 1900–1917"; Anthony Bale, "Women's Toxic Experience"; and Claudia Clark, *Radium Girls: Women and Industrial Health Reform, 1910–1935.*

Political scientists and feminist theorists have examined the implications of industrial poisons and maternity policies on women's employment rights and have generally taken a dim view of efforts to restrict such rights. See Virginia Sapiro, ed., *Women, Biology and Public Policy;* and Sally Kenney, *For Whose Protection? Reproductive Hazards and Exclusionary Policies in the United States and Great Britain.*

Scholarly accounts of women reformers have stressed their activism on behalf of women and children, which some have called a "maternalist" agenda, but historians have not looked carefully at reproductive dangers associated with the workplace, preferring to emphasize the broader risks to family. See, for example, Davis, *American Heroine;*

Barbara Sicherman, "Working It Out: Gender, Profession and Reform in the Career of Alice Hamilton"; Kathryn Kish Sklar, *Florence Kelley and the Nation's Work;* Ellen Fitzpatrick, *Endless Crusade: Women Social Scientists and Progressive Reform;* and Penina Glazer and Miriam Slater, *Unequal Colleagues: The Entrance of Women into the Professions, 1890–1940.*

10. Robert Asher, "Business and Workers' Welfare in the Progressive Era: Workmen's Compensation Reform in Massachusetts, 1880–1911"; Rosner and Markowitz, "Early Movement," 518.

11. George M. Price, "The Employment of Women in Chemical Industries," *Survey* 47 (December 14, 1918): 346.

12. Alice Hamilton, *Exploring the Dangerous Trades: The Autobiography of Alice Hamilton,* 115, 128; Carolyn Malone, "Gender, Work and the State: Government Regulation of Women's Work in the White Lead Trades in England, 1891–1898"; *Boston Transcript,* February 28, 1928, folder 393, box 24, CLM-SL; Joseph C. Aub and Ruth Hapgood, *Pioneer in Modern Medicine: David Linn Edsall of Harvard,* 57; Vilma Hunt, *Work and the Health of Women,* 202; Rosner and Markowitz, "Early Movement," 507.

13. Charles Dickens, *The Uncommercial Traveler—All the Year Round,* cited in Vilma R. Hunt, *Work and the Health of Women,* 201. See also Carolyn Malone, "Gender, Work and the State: Government Regulation of Women's Work in the White Lead Trade in England, 1891–1898."

14. Alice Hamilton, "Women in the Lead Industries," *Bulletin of the Bureau of Labor Statistics,* no. 253 (1919), 5–7; Jeanne M. Stellman and Susan M. Daum, *Work Is Dangerous to Your Health,* 35, 44, 45; Alice Hamilton, "Protection for Women Workers," *Forum* 72 (August 1924): 159.

15. Hamilton, "Women in the Lead Industries," 5–7; *Index Medicus: Catalogue of the Library of the Surgeon-General's Office,* 2d ser., 1900–1919; discussion with Gretchen Worden, Director, Mutter Museum, College of Physicians of Philadelphia, March 1993.

16. Alice Hamilton, "Forty Years in the Poisonous Trades," *American Industrial Hygiene Association Quarterly* 9 (March 1948): 14; Claudia Clark, "The Menace of Benzene: Alice Hamilton and the Health of American Workers," 6; Stellman and Daum, *Work Is Dangerous to Your Health.*

17. Angela Nugent, "The Power to Define a New Disease: Epidemiological Politics and Radium Poisoning," 187; Clark, "The Menace of Benzene," 8.

18. Asher, "Business and Workers' Welfare in the Progressive Era"; David Rosner and Gerald Markowitz, *Deadly Dust: Silicosis and the Politics of Occupational Disease in Twentieth-Century America.*

19. O'Neil Kane, "Unwashed Hands," *Boston Evening Globe,* December 6, 1929; *Sixth Annual Report of the Social Service Department of Massachusetts General Hospital, January 1, 1911 to January 11, 1912,* p. 27, MGH-SSD.

20. Paul Starr, *The Social Transformation of American Medicine: The Rise of a Sovereign Profession and the Making of a Vast Industry,* 200. For information on Taylorism, see Alfred D. Chandler, *The Visible Hand: The Managerial Revolution in American Business.*

21. Morris J. Vogel, *The Invention of the Modern Hospital: Boston, 1870–1930,* 124–5; *Third Annual Report of the Commissioner of Labor and Industry* (Harrisburg: Commonwealth of Pennsylvania, 1916), 32; Aub and Hapgood, *Pioneer in Modern Medicine,* 183; *Pennsylvania Legislative Journal* 5:6581–2; *State of New Jersey Report* (Trenton: Department of Labor, 1912), 3.

22. Robert Watchorn, *Fifth Annual Report of the Factory Inspectors* (Harrisburg: Commonwealth of Pennsylvania, 1894), 455.

23. *Third Annual Report of the Commissioner of Labor and Industry,* 1025–32; *State of New Jersey Report* (1911), 20; *State of New Jersey Report* (1912), 13.

24. "To Make Industry Safe from Poison," *Boston Transcript,* September 4, 1929, folder 393, box 24, CLM-SL; "Woman's Law," *Laws of Pennsylvania* (Harrisburg: Commonwealth of Pennsylvania, 1913), 1028; "Lead Poisoning Law," *Laws of Pennsylvania* (Harrisburg: Commonwealth of Pennsylvania, 1913), 1363.

25. *State of New Jersey Report* (Trenton: Department of Labor, 1913), 3–11; *State of New Jersey Reports,* tuberculosis charts in reports of various years; Rosner and Markowitz, "Early Movement," 512.

26. *State of New Jersey Report* (Trenton: Department of Labor, 1918), 18; Maurine W. Greenwald, *Women, War, and Work: The Impact of World War I on Women Workers in the United States.*

27. Hunt, *Work and the Health of Women,* 202; Rosner and Markowitz, "Early Movement," 507; Alice Hamilton, "The Blanket Amendment—Protection for Women Workers?" *Forum* 72 (August 1924): 159; G. Reid, "Infant Mortality in Relation to Factory Labor," *Transactions of the Thirteenth International Congress on Hygiene and Demography* 3/2 (1912): 943, cited in Anna Baetjer, *Women in Industry: Their Health and Efficiency,* 153; Thomas Oliver, "Industrial Lead Poisoning in Europe," *Bulletin of the Bureau of Labor,* no. 95 (1911). "Germ cells" are the cells in both men and women that contain the genetic material.

28. Oliver, "Industrial Lead Poisoning in Europe," 109; Hamilton, "Women in the Lead Industries," 5–7.

29. Alice Hamilton, "The Lead Industries in the United States," paper presented at International Congress, Brussels, 1912, p. 3, folder 30, box 2, AHP-SL; Hamilton, "Women in the Lead Industries," 11–2; Hamilton, "Possibilities and Limitations," 39.

30. Alice Hamilton, "Lead Poisoning in Potteries, Tile Works, and Porcelain Enameled Sanitary Ware Factories," *Bulletin of the Bureau of Labor,* no. 104 (1912).

31. *Monthly Bulletin of the Pennsylvania Dept. of Labor and Industry* 7/4 (1920): 118, 7/6 (1920): 15; Hamilton, *Exploring the Dangerous Trades,* 130; Thomas Oliver, "Lead Industries in the United States," *Bulletin of the Bureau of Labor,* no. 95 (1911), 112. In a postwar retrospective on the activities of the Industrial Board, one member, Mrs. Samuel Semple, asserted that the board "disapproved, or limited" the employment of women in new occupations when "the material to be handled constitute[d] a special risk for women's physiology greater than that for men." In her detailed report she relied on opinions expressed by medical scientists. See *Monthly Bulletin of the Pennsylvania Department of Labor and Industry* 7/6 (1920): 39.

32. *Preliminary Report of the New York State Factory Investigating Commission* (New York: Department of Labor, 1912), 107.

33. *Preliminary Report of the New York State Factory Investigating Commission,* 483, 500, 300, 503.

34. *Monthly Labor Review* (January 1919): 237.

35. Ibid.

36. Ibid., 238.

37. Alice Hamilton, "The Growing Menace of Benzol Poisoning in American Industry," *Journal of the American Medical Association* 78 (1922): 627–30.

38. Alice Hamilton, "Industrial Poisoning in Making Coal-Tar Dyes and Dye Intermediates," *Bureau of Labor Statistics,* no. 280 (Washington: U.S. Department of Labor, 1921), 6; Alice Hamilton to Florence Kelley, June 5 and May 28, 1924, folder "Correspondence—Dr. Alice Hamilton," reel 26, NCL-LC.

39. Clark, "The Menace of Benzene," 6–9; Alice Hamilton, "Benzene Poisoning in Industry," *The Medical Women's Journal* 38 (September 1931): 221–4; Hamilton, "Forty Years in the Poisonous Trades," 14–5 (with thanks to Dr. Mary Schwanke, Associate Professor of Biology, University of Maine at Farmington, for the physiological explanations). This is not to say, of course, that all proponents of prohibitions against benzene believed that women, especially mothers, belonged in industrial jobs. The actions of the Consumers' League of Massachusetts should be examined because the organization's attention to benzene did not arise from a belief that women belonged in industry. To the contrary, the National Consumers' League stood behind the "Brandeis brief," so influential in the *Muller* decision. The league's interest in working women's health went beyond the biological and was based on women's domestic responsibilities. Members viewed safer working conditions as one step on the road to having women at home with their children full time. The Consumers' League of Massachusetts, for example, opposed day care. See typescript "Charity Flyer" (1929?), folder 49, box 4, CLM-SL.

40. "Occupational Disease," folder 449, box 27, CLM-SL; "Survey Discloses Poisoning among Women Workers," *Boston Sunday Advertiser,* August 4, 1929.

41. Agnes Peterson, "Shoe Industry in New Hampshire," *Bulletin of the Women's Bureau,* no. 121 (1935), 87; "Some Types of Industrial Poisoning: A Bulletin Published by the Consumers' League" (1929?), pp. 3, 6–13, 14, folder 51, box 4, CLM-SL.

42. Alice Hamilton to Florence Kelley, June 5, 1924, and December 8, 1925, folder "Correspondence—Dr. Alice Hamilton," reel 26, NCL-LC.

43. Schedule, "Solvents and Other Substances Used That May Contain Poisons," folder "Schedules (Solvents Used)," box 214, "Women's Bureau Bulletins 1918–1963—No. 121," WB-NA; "A Survey of the Shoe Industry in New Hampshire," *Bulletin of the Women's Bureau,* no. 213 (1935); Bradley Dewey to Alice Hamilton, February 9, 1933, folder 40, box 2, AHP-SL.

44. B. L. Vosburgh (?), Handwritten notes "Case #5912077," folder "Benzol and Compensation," box 1, DIH-NYS; B. L. Vosburgh to Alice Hamilton, 11–2–33, folder 40, box 2, AHP-SL; typed notes "Abstract Case 40106310," folder "Benzol and Compensation," box 1, DIH-NYS.

45. Manfred Bowditch and Henry Elkins, "Chronic Exposure to Benzene," *Journal of Industrial Hygiene and Toxicology* 21 (October 1939): 342.

46. Hunt, *Work and the Health of Women*, 206–7; Claudia Clark, "Glowing in the Dark: The Radium Dial Painters, the Consumers' League and Industrial Health in the United States, 1910–1935." See also Angela Nugent Young, "Alice Hamilton and the Health of American Workers" (Ph.D. diss., Brown University, 1987). For a more complete account of the radium dial painters, see Claudia Clark, *Radium Girls: Women and Industrial Health Reform, 1910–1935* (Chapel Hill: University of North Carolina Press, 1997).

47. Margaret T. Mettert, "The Occurrence and Prevention of Occupational Disease among Women, 1935–1938," *Bulletin of the Women's Bureau*, no. 184 (1941), 29; "Women Workers in Some Expanding Wartime Industries: New Jersey, 1942," box 658, "Women's Bureau Bulletins 1918–1963—no. 197," WB-NA.

48. "Report of Committee on Lead Poisoning," American Public Health Association Meeting, October 1929, 30; Alice Hamilton to Mary van Kleeck, March 19, 1929, folder 248, box 14, MvK-SSC.

49. Ethel Best, "The Employment of Women in Vitreous Enameling," *Bulletin of the Women's Bureau*, no. 101 (1932), viii, 1.

50. Christopher Sellers, "Public Health Service's Office of Industrial Hygiene and the Transformation of Industrial Medicine," 49–53; "Lead Poisoning Law," *Laws of Pennsylvania*, 1364, 1365; "Final Report of the Committee," Chemical and Rubber Sections, National Safety Council (May 1926), folder 42, box 2, AHP-SL.

51. "Conference on Women in Industry," *Special Bulletin of the Pennsylvania Department of Labor and Industry*, no. 10 (1926), 41–80; *State of New Jersey Reports* (Trenton: Department of Labor, 1919–1930).

52. Charles E. Rosenberg, "The Bitter Fruit: Heredity, Disease and Social Thought," 46–9. Rosenberg's *Cholera Years: The United States in 1832, 1849, and 1866*, describes this relationship as well. See also Kessler-Harris, *Out to Work*, 212.

53. Best, "The Employment of Women in Vitreous Enameling," 38; Agnes deLima, "Night-Working Mothers in Textile Mills, Passaic, New Jersey" (Consumers' League of New Jersey, December 1920), folder "Industrial Relations, Pamphlets," box 14, EC-SSC.

Chapter 3

1. Thomas J. O'Brien, "Fatal Case of Lead Poisoning Due to Faulty Personal Hygiene," New York State's *Industrial Hygiene Bulletin* 3/1 (July 1926): 2.

2. Patricia Evridge Hill, "Redefining Occupational Illness: Mill Work, Maternal Health, Social Class and Women's Roles in the Textile South," 3–5. See also Claudia Clark, *Radium Girls: Women and Industrial Health Reform, 1910–1935.*

3. Alice Hamilton and Charles H. Verrill, "Hygiene in the Printing Trades," *Bulletin of the Bureau of Labor Statistics*, no. 209 (April 1917).

4. Susan Porter Benson, *Counter Cultures: Saleswomen, Managers, and Customers in American Department Stores, 1890–1940,* 34, 180.

5. Maud Nathan, *The Story of an Epoch-Making Movement,* 25–8.

6. Ibid., 67. See also Eileen Boris, *Home to Work: Motherhood and the Politics of Industrial Homework in the United States.*

7. Annie S. Daniel, "The Wreck of the Home: How Wearing Apparel Is Fashioned in the Tenements," *Charities* 15 (1905): 624, 628.

8. Susanna P. Zwemer, "History of the Consumers' League of New Jersey (1900–1950)," p. 14 in finding aid, CLNJ-RU.

9. "Behind the Scenes in Candy Factories" (New York: Consumers' League of New York, 1928), pp. 5, 20, 28, 53, 54, folder "Industrial Relations—pamphlets," box 14, EC-SSC.

10. Nathan, *Story of an Epoch-Making Movement,* 74.

11. Josephine Goldmark, *Fatigue and Efficiency: A Study in Industry,* 43, 45, 47, 48; American Telephone and Telegraph, "Welfare Work in Behalf of Telephone Operators" (n.d. [1913?]), pp. 10, 11, 15, 16, folder 332–19, "Industrial Relations—Welfare Work—New York, 1913–1930," box 48, BCC-BL. See also Jill E. Cooper, "Keeping the Girls on the Line: The Medical Department and Women Workers at AT&T, 1913–1940."

12. *New York Herald Tribune,* November 4, 1924.

13. Pamphlet, "The Conference on the Breakdown of Industrial Standards," folder 245, box 15, CLM-SL.

14. See Nancy F. Cott, "What's in a Name? The Limits of 'Social Feminism'; or Expanding the Vocabulary of Women's History," *Journal of American History* 76 (December 1989): 809–29; and Karen Offen, "Deciding Feminism: A Comparative Historical Approach," *Signs* 14 (Autumn 1988).

15. Nancy F. Cott, *The Grounding of Modern Feminism,* 117–42; Wendy Sarvasy, "Beyond the Difference versus Equality Debate: Postsuffrage Feminism, Citizenship, and the Quest for a Feminist Welfare State," *Signs* 17 (Winter 1992): 329–62.

16. "The Work of the Consumers' League of Connecticut" (July 1919), folder 20, box 2, CLC-SL.

17. Kathryn Kish Sklar, "Why Were Most Politically Active Women Opposed to the ERA in the 1920s?" 175–82.

18. *Annual Report of the Industrial Commissioner for the 12 Months Ended June 20, 1926* (Albany: State Department of Labor, 1927), 18; Blanche Wiesen Cook, *Eleanor Roosevelt,* vol. 1: *1884–1933,* 360–1.

19. "U.S. Supreme Court Sustains Law Prohibiting Nightwork by Women in Industry," New York State's *Industrial Bulletin* 3/6 (March 1924): 132.

20. "Reconstruction Explained: Commissioner Shientag Outlines to the State Consumers' League, League of Women Voters, Women's Christian Temperance Union and Allied Organizations the Work of Restoring the Labor Department to Its Former Efficiency," New York State's *Industrial Bulletin* 2/8 (May 1923): 167; "Minimum Wage Law," ibid., 18/6 (June 1939): 258–60.

21. Alice Kessler-Harris, *Out to Work: A History of Wage-Earning Women in the United States,* 209–12.

22. "Health Problems of Women in Industry," *Bulletin of the Women's Bureau,* no. 18 (1921), 8, 9.

23. Rosalie Slaughter-Morton, "Industrial Diseases of Women as a Factor in Eugenics," *Transactions of the Thirty-Ninth Annual Meeting of the Alumni Association of the Woman's Medical College of Pennsylvania* (1914), 77–8.

24. Cott, *Grounding of Modern Feminism,* 129; Mary Anderson to Alice Hamilton, October 8, 1934, folder "Hamilton, Dr. Alice," box 22, General Correspondence of the Women's Bureau, 1918–1948, Office of the Director, WB-NA.

25. "The Employment of Women in Hazardous Industries in the United States," *Bulletin of the Women's Bureau,* no. 6 (1921), 7, 8.

26. "The 48 Hour Week," New York State's *Industrial Bulletin* 6/3 (December 1926): 71; Boris, *Home to Work,* 1–17.

27. National Industrial Conference Board, *Health Services in Industry Report,* no. 34 (New York: National Industrial Conference Board, January 1921), 15. For the early years of industrial medicine, see Paul Starr, *The Social Transformation of American Medicine;* and Morris J. Vogel, *The Invention of the Modern Hospital: Boston, 1870–1930,* 124–5.

28. Barbara Sicherman, *Alice Hamilton: A Life in Letters,* 170.

29. "Notes prepared by Lillian Erskine regarding industrial hygiene in the United States," February 28, 1924, folder 802, box 46, MvK-SSC; Harold Stevens, "The Practice of Medicine in Industry," *New England Journal of Medicine* 203 (November 13, 1930): 974–5; Christopher Sellers, "Public Health Service's Office of Industrial Hygiene and the Transformation of Industrial Medicine," 42–53.

30. Stevens, "The Practice of Medicine in Industry," 975.

31. Richard A. Meckel, *Save the Babies: American Public Health Reform and the Prevention of Infant Mortality, 1850–1929,* 119–20; Alice Hamilton, "The New Public Health—Part I," *Survey* (November 18, 1916): 167.

32. Sellers, "Office of Industrial Hygiene," 63–4; Kenneth Morse and Milton Kronenberg, "Radium Painting: Hazards and Precautions," *Industrial Medicine* 12 (December 1943): 814–7, cited in Clark, "Glowing in the Dark: The Radium Dial Painters, the Consumers' League and Industrial Health in the United States, 1910–1935," 356.

33. "The Medical Examination and Laboratory Tests Made by the Industrial Hygiene Division Favorably Received by Employers and Employees," New York State's *Industrial Hygiene Bulletin* 1/6 (December 1924); Meckel, *Save the Babies,* 91–123.

34. "Health Interviews with 100 Women in the Candy Factory," New York State's *Industrial Bulletin* 5/10 (August 1926): 318. "Dysmenorrhea" is difficult or painful menstruation.

35. David Rosner and Gerald Markowitz, "'A Gift of God'?: The Public Health Controversy over Leaded Gasoline during the 1920s," 126. Note: A threshold-limit

value, or TLV, is the amount of hazardous material in the environment, usually expressed in parts per million, that demarcates a "safe" environment from a potentially unhealthy one.

36. Alice Hamilton, "Industrial Poisons," *New England Journal of Medicine* 209 (August 10, 1933): 279–80.

37. May R. Mayers, "The Compensation Law and Its Application to Lead Cases," New York State's *Industrial Hygiene Bulletin* 5 (October 1928): 13; Mayers, "Clinical and Laboratory Manifestations of Lead Absorption," ibid., (September 1928): 1; Mayers, "Lead Absorption," ibid., (December 1928): 1.

38. Robert Kehoe to May Mayers, December 31, 1943, folder "Lead Committee, American Public Health Association," box 3, DIH-NYS; *Chemical Abstracts* (April 10, 1939), folder "Lead Poisoning #2," box 3, DIH-NYS; *Air Hygiene Federation of America* (September 13, 1939), folder "Lead Poisoning #2," box 3, DIH-NYS; Robert Kehoe to May Mayers, June 10, 1943, folder "Lead Committee, American Public Health Association," box 3, DIH-NYS.

39. May R. Mayers and Minnie M. McMahon, "Industrial Lead Poisoning and Its Prevention," *Special Bulletin* 195 (Albany: New York State Department of Labor, 1938), p. 17, folder "Lead Bulletin Revision," box 3, DIH-NYS; *Air Hygiene Federation of America* (April 22, 1939), folder "Lead Poisoning #2," box 3, DIH-NYS; typescript, R. L. Furney, National Safety Council, "Third Draft of Lead Pamphlet" (September 1940), pp. 11, 17, folder "Lead Poisoning #2," box 3, DIH-NYS. See also Joel Howell, *Technology in the Hospital: Transforming Patient Care in the Early Twentieth Century*.

40. Mary Lakeman, "Menstrual Pain among Industrial Women," *New England Journal of Medicine* 209 (August 3, 1933): 237.

41. Uterine Cancer Cytology Research Project, 1957–1962, Medical College of Pennsylvania Archives and Special Collections on Women in Medicine, Philadelphia; Lakeman, "Menstrual Pain."

42. For more information on the institutionalization of reform agendas, see Alice Kessler-Harris's "Problems of Coalition-Building: Women and the Trade Unions in the 1920s."

43. Committee on Industrial Health, "Health Service in Industry," *New England Journal of Medicine* 222 (February 8, 1940): 241.

44. Nelle Swartz, "The Industrial Nurse," New York State's *Industrial Bulletin* 5/7 (April 1926): 177; "Medical Service in 19 Department Stores," ibid., 7/5 (February 1928): 160. See also Cooper, "Keeping the Girls on the Line," 6.

45. Typescript, "Survey of Company Dispensaries" (n.d.), folder 432, case 2, MRA-BL.

46. Massachusetts Medical Society Committee on Public Education, "Health in Industry," *New England Journal of Medicine* 205 (August 13, 1931): 360–1, and 206 (March 24, 1932): 646.

47. David Rosner and Gerald Markowitz, *Deadly Dust: Silicosis and the Politics of Occupational Disease in Twentieth-Century America*; W. P. Cahill (of Graton and

Knight), "Works Managers Inspection Trip to the Universal Winding Company" (and response), n.d. (1931?), folder 2–13, box 2, MRA-BL; "Survey of Company Dispensaries," folder 432, case 2, MRA-BL.

48. Sellers, "Office of Industrial Hygiene," 52; "Survey of Company Dispensaries," folder 432, case 2, MRA-BL; Doris Stevens, "The Blanket Amendment—A Debate: Suffrage Does Not Give Equality," *Forum* 72 (August 1924): 149.

49. Folder 311–210–19, "New England Industries Surveys—Cotton," pp. 11–2, case 12, BCC-BL; "Some Effects of Legislation Limiting Hours of Work for Women," *Bulletin of the Women's Bureau*, no. 15 (1921); editorial, "The Protection of Women in Industry," *New England Journal of Medicine* 204 (March 12, 1931): 567.

50. Richard Gillespie, *Manufacturing Knowledge: A History of the Hawthorne Experiments* (Cambridge: Cambridge University Press, 1991), 2–3.

51. Ibid., 127–51.

52. Alan Derickson, "Physiological Science and Scientific Management in the Progressive Era: Frederic S. Lee and the Committee on Industrial Fatigue," 497.

53. Margaret T. Mettert, "State Reporting of Occupational Disease, Including a Survey of Legislation Applying to Women," *Bulletin of the Women's Bureau*, no. 114 (1934), 19.

54. Margaret T. Mettert, "The Occurrence and Prevention of Occupational Disease among Women, 1935–1938," *Bulletin of the Women's Bureau*, no. 184 (1941), 15–6; "Women Workers in Some Expanding Wartime Industries: New Jersey, 1942," *Bulletin of the Women's Bureau*, no. 197 (1943), 29–31; Mettert, "Occurrence and Prevention of Occupational Disease," 18–20, 26. Pneumoconiosis is a lung disease caused by prolonged inhalation of metallic dusts.

55. Paul Kellogg to Alice Hamilton, March 15, 1923, folder SWA1 590, reel 26, SA-UML; memorandum, "C.D." to Paul Kellogg, February 25, 1924, folder SWA1 590, reel 26, SA-UML; Alfred E. Shipley to Paul Kellogg, February 27, 1924, folder SWA1 590, reel 26, SA-UML.

Chapter 4

1. Elizabeth Hawes, "Woman War Worker: A Case History," *New York Times Magazine*, December 26, 1943.

2. Ibid.

3. "USES Reports Changing Employer Attitudes," *Employment Security Review* 9 (1942): 12–3; "Women Can Do 80% of War Jobs," *New York Times*, May 23, 1942, folder 1141, box 73, MvK-SSC; Sherna Berger Gluck, *Rosie the Riveter Revisited: Women, the War, and Social Change*, 10; Ruth Milkman, "Redefining 'Women's Work': The Sexual Division of Labor in the Auto Industry during World War II," 216.

4. Tennessee State Board for Vocational Education, "More Efficient Use of Women in Industry, February 1944," pp. 10–1, folder 1–15, box 1, EFW-SSC; Division of Occupational Analysis and Manning Tables, War Manpower Commission, "The Employment of Women: Facing Facts in the Utilization of Manpower" (typescript, June

1943), folder "Council for Defense, 1941," box 190, "Records Re: Women Workers in World War II, 1940–1945," WB-NA; Frank S. Adams, "Women in Democracy's Arsenal," *New York Times Magazine,* October 19, 1941.

5. D'Ann Campbell, *Women at War with America: Private Lives in a Patriotic Era,* 112; Ruth Milkman, "Redefining 'Women's Work,'" 209–22.

6. David Rosner and Gerald Markowitz, *Deadly Dust: Silicosis and the Politics of Occupational Disease in Twentieth-Century America,* 188–9; Anthony Bale, "'Hope in Another Direction': Compensation for Work-Related Illness among Women, 1900–1960," 100.

7. See, for instance, Judith A. Baer, *Chains of Protection: The Judicial Response to Women's Labor Legislation;* Susan Lehrer, *Origins of Protective Labor Legislation for Women, 1905–1925;* Nancy S. Erickson, "*Muller v. Oregon* Reconsidered: The Origins of a Sex-Based Doctrine of Liberty of Contract"; and Alice Kessler-Harris, "The Paradox of Motherhood: Night Work Restrictions in the United States."

8. "Women Speed Jobs in War Factories," *New York Times,* February 14, 1942; Alice Kessler-Harris, *Out to Work: A History of Wage-Earning Women in the United States,* 295–7. See also Lise Vogel, *Mothers on the Job: Maternity Policy in the U.S. Workplace.*

9. Committee on Industrial Health, "Health Problems in Oregon," *Industrial Medicine* 13 (1944): 446.

10. Augusta Clawson, *Shipyard Diary of a Welder* (New York: Penguin Books, 1944), 170; War Manpower Commission Division of Operations—Women's Program, "Employment of Women in Shipyards" (n.d.), folder "Occupations—shipyards," box 202, "Records Re: Women Workers in World War II, 1940–1945," WB-NA; Elinore Herrick, "With Women at Work, the Factory Changes," *New York Times Magazine,* January 24, 1943, p. 34. For male workers' response to physical examinations earlier in the century, see Alan Derickson, "Physiological Science and Scientific Management in the Progressive Era: Frederic S. Lee and the Committee on Industrial Fatigue"; and Angela Nugent, "Organizing Trade Unions to Combat Disease: The Workers' Health Bureau, 1921–1928," *Labor History* 26 (1985): 423–46.

11. F. C. Minaker, "New Jobs for Women—II," *American Business* 12 (1942), folder "Occupation—Ordnance and Explosives—1942," box 201, "Records Re: Women Workers in World War II, 1940–1945," WB-NA; "Put Your Waist Fats in the War Effort," *Marin-er 2* (December 11, 1943), folder 1–15, box 1, EFW-SSC.

12. "Humanizing the Job," *New York Times,* August 8, 1943.

13. "Factory Girl Type Seen Ended by War," *New York Times,* March 23, 1943.

14. "Safety Fashions," National Safety Council, folder "Pamphlets—general," box 16, EC-SSC; "Women Cautioned about War Jobs," *New York Times,* December 13, 1942.

15. Charles-Francis Long, "Women at Work," *Industrial Medicine* 12 (1943): 109.

16. Interview with Juanita Loveless in Gluck, *Rosie the Riveter Revisited,* 136; Herrick, "With Women at Work, the Factory Changes," 33; "Women in Production Work," Monarch Machine Tool Company (n.d), folder "Pamphlets—General," box 16,

Notes to Chapter 4

EC-SSC; Lucy Greenbaum, "I Worked on the Assembly Line," *New York Times Magazine,* March 28, 1943. See also Gluck, *Rosie the Riveter Revisited,* 111, 210.

17. Adams, "Women in Democracy's Arsenal"; "Working Housewives and War Plant Jobs," *New York Times,* September 23, 1944; "New Type of Scraper with Narrow Handle Is Aid to Women Painters," *The Stinger,* August 19, 1944, folder 1–14, box 1, EFW-SSC.

18. "Occupational Analysis, Bath Iron Works, May 8, 1943," folder "Correspondence—1942," box 192, Records Re: Women Workers in World War II, 1940–1945, WB-NA; anonymous (E. F. Ward?), typed summary of experiences, January 7, 1944, folder 1–14, box 1, EFW-SSC; Herrick, "With Women at Work, the Factory Changes."

19. "Women in Production Work"; Nora Stanton Barney, "Women as Human Beings" (published by the author, 1946), pp. 8–9, folder 38, box 2, ALP-SL.

20. William H. Varney, "Medical Management of Complaints of Women in the Explosives Industry," *Industrial Medicine* 13 (1944): 122; Gluck, *Rosie the Riveter Revisited,* 265–7.

21. "Occupational Analysis, Bath Iron Works"; David Kotelchuck, "Asbestos: 'The Funeral Dress of Kings'—and Others," reports that by 1940, the connection between asbestos and lung cancer had attracted the attention of the Public Health Service. But asbestos manufacturers largely controlled the epidemiological data, which they did not generally make available to workers, male or female (see 199–202).

22. Clawson, *Shipyard Diary,* 108, 170. Sherna Berger Gluck's oral histories of wartime women workers echo this notion that accidents "were our own fault."

23. Alice Hamilton to Mary Anderson, January 20, 1941, folder "Correspondence—1941," box 1, Division of Research, Special Bulletins, 1940–1944, WB-NA.

24. Tennessee State Board of Vocational Education, "More Efficient Use of Women in Industry," p. 40; Virginia Lemire to Emma France Ward, August 4, 1944, folder 1–4, box 1, EFW-SSC.

25. O. F. Hedley to P. A. Neal, n.d. (1941?), folder "Correspondence—1941," box 1, Division of Research, Special Bulletins, 1940–1944, WB-NA.

26. Ibid.; Committee on Industrial Health, "Health Problems in Oregon"; Forrest D. Gibson, "Gynecological Examinations in Industry," *Industrial Medicine* 13 (1944): 349.

27. Henry D. Obst, "Plant Use of Chemicals, Poisons, Gases and Related Work Conditions," October 29, 1942, folder "Occupations—Shipyards—1942," box 202, Records Re: Women Workers in World War II, 1940–1945, WB-NA; Marcia L. Patterson, "The History of Marinship's Women in the Crafts, July 1942- July 1945," p. 8, folder 1–12, box 1, EFW-SSC; Margaret Mettert to Mary Anderson, November 17, 1942, folder "Occupations—Shipyards—1942," box 202, Records Re: Women Workers in World War II, 1940–45, WB-NA; Women's Bureau, "Women's Wartime Occupational Hazards," *Industrial Medicine* 12 (1943): 487; Alice Hamilton, "Possibilities and Limitations of the Employment of Women in Industry," *Monthly Bulletin of the Pennsylvania Department of Labor and Industry* 5 (1918): 37, 39.

28. Obst, "Plant Use of Chemicals"; War Manpower Commission Division of Operations, Women's Program, "Employment of Women in Shipyards"; typescript, "Comments on Exposures and Preventive Measures," folder "Occupations—Shipyards—1942," box 202, Records Re: Women Workers in World War II, 1940–45, WB-NA; "Industrial Medicine, North Carolina Shipbuilding Company," September 20, 1943, folder 1–12, box 1, EFW-SSC.

29. Alice Hamilton to Mary Anderson, January 20, 1941, folder "Correspondence—1941," box 1, Division of Research, Special Bulletins, 1940–1944, WB-NA; Alice Hamilton, "Forty Years in the Poisonous Trades," *American Industrial Hygiene Association Quarterly* 9 (1948): 7.

30. National Industrial Information Committee, National Association of Manufacturers "American Women at War" (1942), pp. 32–3, folder "Pamphlets—General," box 16, EC-SSC.

31. Milton Kronenberg, "Working Conditions of Female Employees," *Journal of the American Medical Association* 124 (1944): 677, 681.

32. Max Burnell, "Gynecological and Obstetrical Problems of the Industrial Physician," *Industrial Medicine* 13 (1944): 211–4; A. C. Dick, H. E. Billig, Jr., and H. N. Macy, "Menstrual Exercises," *Industrial Medicine* 12 (1943): 588; H. Close Hesseltine, "Specific Problems of Women in Industry," *Journal of the American Medical Association* 124 (1944): 695; C. O. Sappington, "Health Problems of Women in Industry," *Industrial Medicine* 12 (1943): 215.

33. W. A. Sawyer, quoted in the discussion following Frank A. Barlow, "Proper Placement of Women in Industry," *Journal of the American Medical Association* 124 (1944): 691; "Letters to the Editor," *New York Times Magazine,* October 19, 1941.

34. *Marin-er 2* (December 11, 1943), folder 1–15, box 1, EFW-SSC; California Shipbuilding Corporation to Emma France Ward, November 14, 1943, folder 1–11, box 1, EFW-SSC; "Employing Women in Shipyards," *Bulletin of the Women's Bureau,* no. 192-6 (1944), 23–5.

35. Tennessee State Board of Vocational Education, "More Efficient Use of Women in Industry," 46; Hawes, "Woman War Worker."

36. Josephine Goldmark, *Fatigue and Efficiency: A Study in Industry;* Alan Derickson, "Physiological Science"; Richard Gillespie, *Manufacturing Knowledge: A History of the Hawthorne Experiments; Victory Fleet,* January 1, 1945, p. 4, folder 1–14, box 1, EFW-SSC.

37. Campbell, *Women at War with America,* 131–3; Josephine Newman, "Employing Women in Shipyards," *Bulletin of the Women's Bureau,* no. 192-6 (1944), 40; "Employment of Women in Army Supply Depots in 1943," *Bulletin of the Women's Bureau,* no. 192-8 (1945).

38. Mildred Davis to Emma France Ward, April 26, 1945, folder 1–14, box 1, EFW-SSC. See a variety of reports and letters from the Emma France Ward Papers, including Ilene Sullivan, "Employment of Women and Counseling at Walter Butler Shipbuilding, Inc.," and Patterson, "The History of Marinship's Women in the Crafts, July 1942—July 1945," both in folder 1–12, box 1. See also Virginia Lemire to Emma

France Ward, August 4, 1944; Lillian Angell to Emma France Ward, November 13, 1944; Mildred Davis to Emma France Ward, April 26, 1945; and Addie Bishop to Emma France Ward, March 13, 1945, all in folder 1–4, box 1, EFW-SSC.

39. Virginia Lemire to Emma France Ward, August 4, 1944, folder 1–4, box 1, EFW-SSC; "Analysis of Female Absenteeism in an East Coast Shipyard" (n.d.), folder 1–12, box 1, EFW-SSC; Virginia Lemire to J. O. Murray et al., December 28, 1944, folder 1–12, box 1, EFW-SSC; Gluck, *Rosie the Riveter Revisited,* 249.

40. Marcia Patterson, "Why 'Gals' Take Off," *The Stinger,* January 22, 1944, folder 1–14, box 1, EFW-SSC; Gluck, *Rosie the Riveter Revisited,* 249.

41. Tennessee State Board of Vocational Education, "More Efficient Use of Women in Industry," 11–7.

42. Lemire to Murray et al., December 28, 1944.

43. Both Nancy Gabin, in her study of women auto workers (*Feminism in the Labor Movement: Women and the United Auto Workers, 1935–1975),* and Dorothy Sue Cobble, in her work on waitresses, "Recapturing Working-Class Feminism: Union Women in the Postwar Era," have observed the tension between equality and difference among women workers that developed in the postwar period.

Chapter 5

1. Alice Hamilton to Elizabeth A. Magee, May 15, 1953, folder "IV.W–14 Equal Rights—Correspondence, 1953," reel 52, NCL-LC.

2. Alice Hamilton, "Women Workers and Industrial Poisons," *Bulletin of the Women's Bureau,* no. 57 (1926), 2–3.

3. Alice Hamilton, "Possibilities and Limitations of the Employment of Women in Industry," *Monthly Bulletin of the Pennsylvania Department of Labor and Industry* 5/1 (1918).

4. Nancy F. Cott, *The Grounding of Modern Feminism.*

5. Ibid., 117–42. Historians of feminism and of social welfare have begun to delineate the complex relationship that belied these oppositional views. The political scientist Wendy Sarvasy has argued that the sharp public division over the ERA complicated and sometimes worked against feminists' common agenda of gender equality within a construct of gender differentiation. With respect to protective legislation, historians have found real differences over the responsibility for health and the definition of "protection," but some agreement over other issues (Wendy Sarvasy, "Beyond the Difference versus Equality Debate: Postsuffrage Feminism, Citizenship and the Quest for a Feminist Welfare State").

6. Ada R. Wolff, "Women in Industry," pamphlet, box 14, folder "Employment Collection—Industrial Relations," EC-SSC; "Proceedings of the Women's Industrial Conference," *Bulletin of the Women's Bureau,* no. 33 (1926), 53–4.

7. Cott, *The Grounding of Modern Feminism,* 125; M. Carey Thomas to Mary Anderson, February 5, 1924, folder 4, Mary Anderson Collection, Schlesinger Library, Radcliffe College, Harvard University Libraries, Cambridge, Massachusetts.

8. Agnes deLima, "Night-Working Mothers in Textile Mills, Passaic, New Jersey," pamphlet (December 1920), p. 13, folder "Industrial Relations—pamphlets," box 14, EC-SSC.

9. Alice Hamilton to Florence Kelley, April 5, 1924, folder "Correspondence—Dr. Alice Hamilton," reel 26, NCL-LC; "Meeting of the Board of Directors, Monday, June 9, 9:30 A.M.," pp. 2–3, box 59, folder 3037 1–6, part 1, AMWA-MCP.

10. "The Tenth Annual Meeting of the Medical Women's National Association, held at Hotel Sherman, Chicago, June 8, 9, 10, 1924," pp. 79–80, box 59, folder 3037 1–6, part 2, AMWA-MCP; "Wages and Hours Bill," *Medical Women's Journal* 45 (January 1938): 18; Elizabeth A. Magee to Alice Hamilton, October 26, 1944, folder "Correspondence—Dr. Alice Hamilton," reel 26, NCL-LC.

11. Josephine Goldmark, *Fatigue and Efficiency: A Study in Industry*, 95; "Proceedings of the Women's Industrial Conference," *Bulletin of the Women's Bureau*, no. 33 (1926), 32.

12. New York State Factory Investigating Commission, *Preliminary Report* (New York: State Department of Labor, 1913), 261–2; Alice Kessler-Harris, *Out to Work: A History of Wage-Earning Women in the United States*, 204.

13. "English Women Up in Arms," *Medical Women's Journal* 34 (March 1927): 85.

14. Frances Perkins, "Do Women in Industry Need Protection?" *Survey* 55 (February 15, 1926): 531.

15. Elizabeth Faulkner Baker, "Do Women in Industry Need Protection?" *Survey* 55 (February 15, 1926): 583.

16. Leila Rupp and Verta Taylor, *Survival in the Doldrums: The American Women's Rights Movement, 1945 to the 1960s;* Cott, *The Grounding of Modern Feminism*, 121; Doris Stevens, "The Blanket Amendment—A Debate: Suffrage Does Not Give Equality," *Forum* 72 (August 1924): 148; "Meeting of the Board of Directors, Monday, June 9, 9:30 A.M.," pp. 2–3; Sarvasy, "Beyond the Difference versus Equality Debate."

17. Hamilton, "Possibilities and Limitations," 39.

18. "Lost Time and Labor Turnover in Cotton Mills," *Bulletin of the Women's Bureau*, no. 52 (1926); "Employment of Women at Night," *Bulletin of the Women's Bureau*, no. 64 (1928); Lucy Randolph Macon, "Standards for Workers in Southern Industry" (November 1931), p. 27, folder "Industrial Relations," box 14, EC-SSC.

19. Goldmark, *Fatigue and Efficiency*, 95–6.

20. Mary Ryan, *Womanhood in America: From Colonial Times to the Present*, 305–14; Claudia Goldin, *Understanding the Gender Gap: An Economic History of American Women*, 189–98.

21. Alice Hamilton, "Protection for Women Workers," *Forum* 72 (August 1924): 152, 159.

22. Alice Kessler-Harris, "Problems of Coalition-building: Women and Trade Unions in the 1920s," 116–8; Stevens, "The Blanket Amendment," 149.

23. Charles E. Rosenberg, "The Therapeutic Revolution: Medicine, Meaning, and Social Change in Nineteenth-Century America." See also Stanley Joel Reiser, *Medicine and the Reign of Technology*.

24. Doris Stevens, "The Blanket Amendment," 149.

25. "Tenth Annual Meeting of the Medical Women's National Association," pp. 73–8; Hamilton, "Possibilities and Limitations," 37.

26. Alice Hamilton, *Exploring the Dangerous Trades: The Autobiography of Alice Hamilton,* 146.

27. Barbara Sicherman, *Alice Hamilton: A Life in Letters,* 296–303.

28. Alice Hamilton to Florence Kelley, May 28, 1924, folder "Correspondence—Dr. Alice Hamilton," reel 26, NCL-LC.

29. Christopher Sellers, "The Public Health Service's Office of Industrial Hygiene and the Transformation of Industrial Medicine," 52–3.

30. Hamilton, "Protection for Women Workers," 156.

31. Lillian Symes, "Behind the Scenes in Candy Factories," Consumers' League of New York pamphlet (1928), p. 49, folder "Industrial Relations," box 14, EC-SSC.

32. Agnes deLima, "Night-Working Mothers," pp. 11–3.

33. Alice Hamilton, "Women in the Lead Industries," *Bulletin of the Bureau of Labor Statistics,* no. 253 (1919), 12; Richard A. Meckel, *Save the Babies: American Public Health Reform and the Prevention of Infant Mortality, 1850–1929.*

34. Hamilton, "Women in the Lead Industries," 5–7; Jeanne M. Stellman and Susan M. Daum, *Work Is Dangerous to Your Health;* Hamilton, "Protection for Women Workers," 159; Sicherman, *Alice Hamilton,* 254.

35. "Tenth Annual Meeting of the Medical Women's National Association," pp. 76–8.

36. Allen F. Davis, *American Heroine: The Life and Legend of Jane Addams;* Judith Walzer Leavitt, *The Healthiest City: Milwaukee and the Politics of Health Reform;* John Duffy, "Social Impact of Disease in the Late Nineteenth Century"; Sicherman, *Alice Hamilton.*

37. See, for instance, Leavitt, *Healthiest City;* Meckel, *Save the Babies;* and Naomi Rogers, *Dirt and Disease: Polio before FDR.* For an interpretation of more recent public health battles, see Randy Shilts, *And the Band Played On: Politics, People, and the AIDS Epidemic.*

38. Alice Hamilton and Gertrude Seymour, "The New Public Health—III," *Survey* (April 21, 1917): 59–62.

39. "Charity Flyer," typescript (1929?), folder 49, CLM-SL. See Rosner and Markowitz, *Deadly Dust,* on silicosis; Alice Hamilton, "Benzene Poisoning in Industry," *Medical Women's Journal* 38 (September 1931): 221–4, on benzene; and May R. Mayers, "Clinical and Laboratory Manifestations of Lead Absorption," New York State's *Industrial Hygiene Bulletin* 5 (September 1928) on lead. See also "Health Problems of Women in Industry," *Bulletin of the Women's Bureau,* no. 18 (1921), 2 (reprint of May 1921 article in *The Nation's Health*); Hamilton, "Protection for Working Women," *The Woman Citizen* (March 8, 1924): 8. For evidence of attitudes expressed by the Consumers' League of Massachusetts, see papers in CLM-SL.

40. Kessler-Harris, "Problems of Coalition-Building," 110–38; Kathryn Kish Sklar, "Why Were Most Politically Active Women Opposed to the ERA in the 1920s?"

41. Alice Hamilton to Frieda Miller, January 18, 1945, folder "Hamilton, Dr. Alice," box 22, General Correspondence of the Women's Bureau, 1919–1948, WB-NA; Alice Hamilton to Mary Anderson, January 29, 1941, folder "Correspondence—1941," box 1, Division of Research, Special Bulletins, 1940–44, WB-NA.

42. Alice Hamilton to Elizabeth A. Magee, May 30, 1944, and Elizabeth Magee to Alice Hamilton, October 26, 1944, both in folder "Correspondence—Dr. Alice Hamilton," reel 26, NCL-LC.

43. Alice Hamilton, "Why I Am *Against* the Equal Rights Amendment," *Ladies' Home Journal* (July 1945), 123.

44. Ibid., 123.

45. Alice Hamilton, "Forty Years in the Poisonous Trades," *American Industrial Hygiene Association Quarterly* 9 (March 1948): 7.

46. Ibid.; Elizabeth Magee to Alice Hamilton, April 21, 1947, and Alice Hamilton to Elizabeth Magee, April 24, 1947, both in folder "Correspondence—Dr. Alice Hamilton," reel 26, NCL-LC.

47. Alice Hamilton to Elizabeth Magee, August 24, 1945, and Elizabeth Magee to Alice Hamilton, September 7, 1945, both in folder "Correspondence—Dr. Alice Hamilton," reel 26, NCL-LC; Alice Hamilton to Florence Kitchelt, May 17, 1952, cited in Sicherman, *Alice Hamilton,* 385.

48. Alice Hamilton to Elizabeth Magee, May 15, 1953, folder "IV.W–14 Equal Rights—Correspondence, 1953," reel 52, NCL-LC.

49. Hamilton, "Forty Years in the Poisonous Trades," 7.

50. Alice Hamilton to Elizabeth Magee, May 28, 1953, and Alice Hamilton to Elizabeth Magee, May 15, 1953, both in folder "IV.W–14 Equal Rights—Correspondence, 1953," reel 52, NCL-LC.

51. "Women's Bureau Withdraws Opposition," *Equal Rights* (October 1954), folder "IV.W–14 Equal Rights—Correspondence, 1954–1957," reel 52, NCL-LC; Kessler-Harris, *Out to Work,* 306–7.

Chapter 6

1. Standard Oil of New Jersey, "The Worker's Private Woes," *The Medical Bulletin (Doctors in Oil)* 14 (October 1954): 56–7, folder 3, box 82, Series 4 Grants, RBF-RAC.

2. Jean Spencer Felton, "Industrial Health as a Specialty: A Medical Field of Interest to Women Physicians," *Journal of the American Medical Women's Association* 2 (1947): 295–6; Jimmy Pinkston, "Industrial Health: Conversion and Expansion," *Journal of the American Medical Women's Association* 2 (1947): 274.

3. Samuel L. H. Burk, "Management, Medicine and the Future," in pamphlet "Industrial Health: Its Contribution to the Health of a Nation" (Philadelphia: Occupational Health Institute, 1956), p. 21, folder 3, box 82, Series 4 Grants, RBF-RAC; Katharine Boucot, "Detection of Chest Disease—by Survey Methods," *Industrial Medicine and Surgery* 25 (November 1956): 530–2, box 7, KBS-MCP.

4. The papers of Dr. Katharine Sturgis contain numerous articles on her work on

tuberculosis and lung cancer among male workers. These are located primarily in box 7, labeled "Reprints 1943–1963," and include Katharine Boucot Sturgis, "Workers as Populations for Study," *AMA Archives of Environmental Health* (December 1967); records of the Uterine Cancer Cytology Research Project, 1957–1962, Medical College of Pennsylvania Pathology Department, Medical College of Pennsylvania Archives and Special Collections on Women in Medicine, Philadelphia.

5. David Rosner and Gerald Markowitz, *Deadly Dust: Silicosis and the Politics of Occupational Disease in Twentieth-Century America*, 179, 188–90.

6. Alice Hamilton to Frieda Miller, January 18, 1945, folder "Hamilton, Dr. Alice," box 22, General Correspondence of the Women's Bureau, 1919–1948, WB-NA; Massachusetts's "Rules Relating to the Employment of Women," *Industrial Bulletin* (Massachusetts Department of Labor and Industry), no. 10 (1940), sections 28–9.

7. Alice Hamilton to Elizabeth Magee, November 25, 1944, folder "Correspondence—Dr. Alice Hamilton," reel 26, NCL-LC.

8. Nora Stanton Barney, "Women as Human Beings" (published by the author, 1946), pp. 8–9, folder 38, box 2, ALP-SL.

9. Alice Kessler-Harris, *Out to Work: A History of Wage-Earning Women in the United States*, 306, 308, 310.

10. Margaret Mettert, "State Reporting of Occupational Disease, Including a Survey of Legislation Applying to Women," *Bulletin of the Women's Bureau*, no. 114 (1934), 5, 38–9.

11. Mary Anderson to Elizabeth Magee, February 7, 1955, folder "IV.W–14 Equal Rights—Correspondence, 1954–1957," reel 52, NCL-LC.

12. Gerda Seidelin Wegener to MWIA Executive Committee, September 20, 1948, folder "VI Congress: Philadelphia—1950," box 2, MWIA-MCP.

13. Ibid.; Germaine Montreuil-Straus to Gerda Seidelin Wegener, October 12, 1948; Wegener to Montreuil-Straus, January 6, 1949; Wegener to Maria Teresa Casassa, January 6, 1949, all in folder "VI Congress: Philadelphia—1950," box 2, MWIA-MCP.

14. Germaine Montreuil-Straus to Gerda Seidelin Wegener, November 3, 1948, and Wegener to Casassa, January 6, 1949, folder "VI Congress: Philadelphia—1950," box 2, MWIA-MCP.

15. Gerda Seidelin, "Pathology and Hygiene of Housework," *Journal of the American Medical Women's Association* 6 (January 1951): 24; Inger Haldorsen, "Medical Aspects of Housework," *Journal of the American Medical Women's Association* 8 (May 1953): 178; Esther Puhl Lovejoy and Ada Chree Reid, notebook "Medical Women's International Association: An Historical Sketch, 1919–1950," box 58, MWIA-MCP.

16. Zaida Ericksson-Lihr, "Medical Aspects of Housework," *Journal of the American Medical Women's Association* 8 (February 1953): 58; Lovejoy and Reid, "An Historical Sketch," pp. 29–38, box 58, MWIA-MCP.

17. Ruth Geri Hagy, "Cheer Up, Housewife—You're in Much Better Shape Than You Think," *Philadelphia Sunday Bulletin*, September 17, 1950.

18. Minutes of the Board of Directors, January 9, 1947—March 31, 1950, folder 6, box 1, CLC-SL. See also Kessler-Harris, *Out to Work*, 306.

19. Typescript, "State Regulations of the Uses of Radioactive Materials," folder "National Consumers' League—Radiation—Proposed Conference, 1962," reel 84, NCL-LC.

20. Ibid.

21. Ned Parsekian, testimony before Joint Committee on Atomic Energy, March 18, 1959, and "Policy Statement of Board of Directors on Protection of Workers against Radiation Hazards and Recommended Legislation," n.d. [1959], both in folder "National Consumers League—Radiation—1959—Committee Corres., Special Committee on Radiation Exposure," reel 85, NCL-LC.

22. Claudia Clark, "Glowing in the Dark: The Radium Dial Painters, the Consumers' League and Industrial Health in the United States, 1910–1935."

23. Vera Mayer to Susanna Zwemer, n.d. [1959], folder "National Consumers League—Radiation—1959—Committee Corres., Special Committee on Radiation Exposure," reel 85, NCL-LC.

24. Susanna Zwemer to Elizabeth Magee, June 20, 1959, folder "National Consumers League—Radiation—1959—Committee Corres., Special Committee on Radiation Exposure," reel 85, NCL-LC; Harriet L. Hardy, "Medical Progress: Occupational Medicine," *New England Journal of Medicine* 247 (September 25 and October 2, 1952): 473–83, 515–24; Seward E. Miller "The Metamorphosis of Occupational Medicine to Environmental Medicine," *Archives of Environmental Health* 11 (December 1965): 856–7.

25. Lynne Page Snyder, "'The Death-Dealing Smog over Donora, Pennsylvania': Industrial Air Pollution, Public Health, and Federal Policy, 1915–1963."

26. Katharine Boucot Sturgis, "The Driftwood Case: Pioneering Antipollution in Pennsylvania," *Transactions and Studies (of the College of Physicians of Philadelphia)* 14 (December 1982); Katharine Boucot and Doris Freudenberg, "Health Status of Residents of Driftwood, Pennsylvania," typescript, box 15, "Driftwood Case, Asbestos Case, etc.," KBS-MCP; Katharine Sturgis, "Air Pollution and Health," speech presented at the February 26, 1968, meeting of the Lackawanna County Medical Society, Scranton, Pennsylvania, box 5, KBS-MCP.

27. Boucot and Freudenberg, "Health Status of Residents of Driftwood, Pennsylvania"; Sturgis, "Air Pollution and Health"; Katharine Boucot, "Driftwood Case, Asbestos Case, etc.," undated holograph, box 15, KBS-MCP.

28. My thanks to Patricia Reeve, University of Massachusetts, Boston, for this analogy.

29. Interview with Katharine Sturgis, M.D., Oral History Project on Women in Medicine, Medical College of Pennsylvania Archives and Special Collections on Women in Medicine, Philadelphia, 75–6; Nancy Yanes Hoffman, "Katharine Sturgis, M.D.," *Journal of the American Medical Association* 238 (November 28, 1977): 2345.

30. Rachel Carson, *Silent Spring*.

31. Ibid.; Lewis Herber, *Our Synthetic Environment;* René Dubos, "The Conflict between Progress and Safety," *Archives of Environmental Health* 6 (July–December 1963): 12.

32. Katharine Sturgis, "Introductory Remarks: Goals of the Conference," *Journal of Occupational Medicine* 15 (1973), box 8, KBS-MCP; Katharine Sturgis to Willard Sterne Randall, July 17, 1976, box 4, KBS-MCP; Dick Aarons, "Low-Level Pollution: Nuisance or Danger?" *Philadelphia Daily News,* March 23, 1967.

33. *Health and Safety Bulletin* 4 (April 1969), folder "Health and Safety Bulletins 66—April 69," box 88, International Union of Electrical Workers Records (partially processed), Rutgers University Libraries, New Brunswick.

34. John A. Zapp, "Industry and Environmental Health," *Archives of Environmental Health* 9 (November 1964): 684.

Chapter 7

1. Ruth Rosen, "What Feminist Victory in the Court?" *New York Times,* April 1, 1991, A:32.

2. Alice Hamilton, "Women in the Lead Industries," *Bulletin of the Bureau of Labor Statistics,* no. 253 (1919); *Pat L. Grant v. General Motors Corporation, et al.,* 743 F.Supp. 1260 (N.D. Ohio, 1989).

3. *Grant v. General Motors.*

4. Thomas Oliver, "Industrial Lead Poisoning in Europe," *Bulletin of the Bureau of Labor,* no. 95 (1911); Jeanne M. Stellman and Susan M. Daum, *Work Is Dangerous to Your Health;* May Mayers, "The Treatment of Lead Poisoning," New York State's *Industrial Hygiene Bulletin* 3 (November 1926): 1.

5. Anna M. Baetjer, "The Relation of Industrial Work to Obstetrical and Gynecologic Conditions," *Journal of the American Medical Women's Association* 2 (1947): 277.

6. G. Vermande-Van Eck and J. W. Meigs, "Changes in the Ovary of the Rhesus Monkey after Chronic Lead Intoxication," *Fertility and Sterility* 11 (1960): 223, cited in Hunt, *Work and the Health of Women,* 99.

7. Alice Hamilton, "Protection for Women Workers?" *Forum* 72 (August 1924): 159; Oliver, "Industrial Lead Poisoning in Europe," 109; Hamilton, "Women in the Lead Industries," 5–7.

8. David Rosner and Gerald Markowitz, *Deadly Dust: Silicosis and the Politics of Occupational Disease in Twentieth-Century America,* 83–6.

9. *Dietrich v. Northampton,* 138 Mass. (1884); *Bonbrest v. Kotz,* 65 F.Supp. 138 (1946); "Court Backs Right of Women to Jobs with Health Risks," *New York Times,* March 21, 1991, A:1. See also Robert Blank, *Fetal Protection in the Workplace: Women's Rights, Business Interests, and the Unborn;* and Cynthia R. Daniels, *At Women's Expense: State Power and the Politics of Fetal Rights.*

10. Locke Litton Mackenzie, "Compensable Gynecological and Obstetrical Conditions in Women in Industry," *Compensation Medicine* 4 (September–November 1952): 3–7.

11. Rosner and Markowitz, *Deadly Dust,* 179–90.

12. Standard Oil of New Jersey, "The Worker's Private Woes," *The Medical Bulletin (Doctors in Oil)* 14 (October 1954): 56, folder 3, box 82, Series 4 Grants, RBF-RAC.

13. Ida Cannon, *On the Social Frontier of Medicine: Pioneering in Medical Social Service;* Regina Kunzel, *Fallen Women, Problem Girls: Unmarried Mothers and the Professionalization of Social Work, 1890–1945.* See also Mazie Hough, "'I'm a Poor Girl in Family and I Want to Know If You Be Kind': The Community's Response to Unwed Mothers in Maine and Tennessee, 1876–1954."

14. "Women's Bureau Withdraws Opposition," *Equal Rights* (October 1954), folder "IV.W–14 Equal Rights—Correspondence, 1954–1957," reel 52, NCL-LC. Also, see Women's Bureau *Bulletins*, published by the U.S. Department of Labor, beginning in 1950.

15. Alice Hamilton, "Forty Years in the Poisonous Trades," *American Industrial Hygiene Association Quarterly* 9 (March 1948): 7; Alice Hamilton to Elizabeth Magee, September 7, 1945, NCL-LC.

16. Nora Stanton Barney, "Women as Human Beings" (published by the author, 1946), pp. 9, 10, folder 38, box 2, ALP-SL; Mackenzie, "Compensable Gynecological and Obstetrical Conditions"; J. Whitridge Williams, *Obstetrics,* 4th ed. (New York: D. Appleton, 1917); Leila J. Rupp and Verta Taylor, *Survival in the Doldrums: The American Women's Rights Movement, 1945 to the 1960s,* 7.

17. Baetjer, "Relation of Industrial Work to Obstetrical and Gynecologic Conditions," 277.

18. "Court Backs Right of Women to Jobs with Health Risks."

19. Nancy F. Gabin, *Feminism in the Labor Movement: Women and the United Auto Workers, 1935–1975,* 181; Dorothy Sue Cobble, "Recapturing Working-Class Feminism: Union Women in the Postwar Era," in *Not June Cleaver: Women and Gender in Postwar America, 1945–1960,* ed. Joanne Meyerowitz (Philadelphia: Temple University Press, 1994), 73.

20. Hamilton, "Forty Years in the Poisonous Trades," 8; Rosner and Markowitz, *Deadly Dust,* 203–4; David Kotelchuck, "Asbestos: 'The Funeral Dress of Kings'—and Others," 192–207.

21. Reuben Cares, "Thesaurosis from Inhaled Hair Spray?" *Archives of Environmental Health* 11 (July 1965): 80, 86; Om P. Sharma and M. Henry Williams, Jr., "Thesaurosis: Pulmonary Function Studies in Beauticians," *Archives of Environmental Health* 13 (November 1966): 616–8.

22. Council for Occupational Health, "Occupational Health Services for Women Employees," *Archives of Environmental Health* 3 (October 1961): 69–73.

23. Sara Evans, *Born for Liberty: A History of Women in America,* 292–4.

24. Ibid.; Jeanne Mager Stellman, *Women's Work, Women's Health: Myths and Realities,* 179; Kristen Luker, *Abortion and the Politics of Motherhood,* 62–5.

25. Interview with Katharine Sturgis, M.D., Oral History Project on Women in Medicine, Medical College of Pennsylvania Archives and Special Collections on Women in Medicine. See also Regina Markell Morantz-Sanchez, *Sympathy and Science: Women Physicians in American Medicine.*

26. Gabin, *Feminism in the Labor Movement;* Lisa Kannenberg, "'Is Mommy Hav-

ing a Speed-Up Too?' GE, UE, and Representations of Women in the Postwar Workplace," paper presented at the annual meeting of the Organization of American Historians, March 1995.

27. Evans, *Born for Liberty,* 272–6.

28. *Margaret Liddy v. Fisher Body, GM, Pontiac* (filed November 9 and December 31, 1965); *Marjorie Stanchak v. Screw and Bolt Corporation of America* (filed February 8, 1966); Marjorie D. Tibbs to Herman Edelsberg, June 8, 1966; Herman Edelsberg to Charles Duncan, July 5, 1966, folder "Sex decisions," box 295, International Union of Electrical Workers Records (partially processed), Rutgers University Libraries, New Brunswick, New Jersey.

29. Lise Vogel, *Mothers on the Job: Maternity Policy in the U.S. Workplace,* 57; Nancy F. Cott, *The Grounding of Modern Feminism,* 134–42.

30. Vogel, *Mothers on the Job,* 79, 91–113.

31. Ibid., 63. Vogel notes that this separation was a new strategy.

32. Vilma Hunt, "Work and the Health of Women," folder 126, box 7, HLH-SL.

33. Andrea M. Hricko and Cora Baglet Marrett, "Women's Occupational Health: The Rise and Fall of a Research Issue," p. 8, folder 126, box 7, HLH-SL.

34. David Wegman, "Occupational Health Hazards of Women," p. 7, folder 126, box 7, HLH-SL.

35. Stellman, *Women's Work, Women's Health,* 179.

36. OTA, *Reproductive Health Hazards,* 264; Phyllis Lehmann, "Women Workers: Are They Special?" *Job Safety and Health* 3 (April 1975): 12.

37. OTA, *Reproductive Health Hazards,* 264–5.

38. Ibid., 251.

39. Sally J. Kenney, *For Whose Protection? Reproductive Hazards and Exclusionary Policies in the United States and Great Britain; International Union, United Automobile Workers v. Johnson Controls, Inc.,* 111 S.Ct. 1196 (1991); "Court Backs Right of Women to Jobs With Health Risks."

Epilogue

1. Amrita Basu, *The Challenge of Local Feminisms: Women's Movements in Global Perspective,* 17, 14; Marguerite Guzman Bouvard, *Revolutionizing Motherhood: The Mothers of the Plaza de Mayo;* Karen J. Hossfeld, "'Their Logic against Them': Contradictions in Sex, Race, and Class in Silicon Valley," 149–78; Emily Martin, *The Woman in the Body: A Cultural Analysis of Reproduction,* 113–38.

2. Lesley Doyal, *What Makes Women Sick: Gender and the Political Economy of Health,* 223.

3. Ruth Rosen, "What Feminist Victory in the Court?" *New York Times,* April 1, 1991, A:32; Sally Kenney, *For Whose Protection? Reproductive Hazards and Exclusionary Policies in the United States and Great Britain;* Cynthia R. Daniels, *At Women's Expense:*

State Power and the Politics of Fetal Rights; Lise Vogel, *Mothers on the Job: Maternity Policy in the United States.*

4. Peter T. Kilborn, "Who Decides Who Works at Jobs Imperiling Fetuses?" *New York Times,* September 2, 1990.

5. Linda Gordon, "The New Feminist Scholarship on the Welfare State."

6. Rebecca Mead, "Eggs for Sale"; Janet Golden, "Creating FAS, or: Doctors Can Discover Disease but It Takes a Whole Society to Make a Syndrome."

Bibliography

Amoskeag Manufacturing Company Papers. Baker Library Manuscripts and Special Collections, Harvard University Libraries. Cambridge, Massachusetts.

Mary Anderson Collection. Schlesinger Library, Radcliffe College, Harvard University Libraries. Cambridge, Massachusetts.

Apple, Rima, ed. *Women, Health, and Medicine: A Historical Handbook*. New York: Garland, 1990.

Asher, Robert. "Business and Workers' Welfare in the Progressive Era: Workmen's Compensation Reform in Massachusetts, 1880–1911." *Business History Review* 43 (Winter 1969): 452–75.

Aub, Joseph C., and Ruth Hapgood. *Pioneer in Modern Medicine: David Linn Edsall of Harvard*. Cambridge: Harvard Medical Alumni Association, 1970.

Baer, Judith. *Chains of Protection: The Judicial Response to Women's Labor Legislation*. Westport, Conn.: Greenwood Press, 1978.

Baetjer, Anna. *Women in Industry: Their Health and Efficiency*. Baltimore: Johns Hopkins University Press, 1946.

Bale, Anthony. "Women's Toxic Experience." In *Women, Health, and Medicine in America: A Historical Handbook*, ed. Rima Apple. New York: Garland, 1990.

———. "'Hope in Another Direction': Compensation for Work-Related Illness among Women, 1900–1960." Parts 1 and 2. *Women and Health* 15 (1989): 81–102, 99–115.

Barlow, Alfred. *The History and Principles of Weaving by Hand and by Power*. Boston: Sampson, Law, Martson, Searle, and Rivington, 1884.

Basu, Amrita, ed. *The Challenge of Local Feminisms: Women's Movements in Global Perspective*. Boulder, Colo.: Westview Press, 1995.

Bell, Carolyn. "Implementing Safety and Health Regulations for Women in the Workplace." *Feminist Studies* 5 (Summer 1979): 286–301.

Benson, Susan Porter. *Counter Cultures: Saleswomen, Managers and Customers in American Department Stores, 1890–1940*. Urbana: University of Illinois Press, 1988.

Berebitsky, Julie. "'Like' Our Very Own: Adoptive Parenthood in the United States, 1870–1945." Ph.D. diss., Temple University, 1997.

Blank, Robert. *Fetal Protection in the Workplace: Women's Rights, Business Interests, and the Unborn*. New York: Columbia University Press, 1993.

Boris, Eileen. *Home to Work: Motherhood and the Politics of Industrial Homework in the United States*. Cambridge: Cambridge University Press, 1994.

Bouvard, Marguerite Guzman. *Revolutionizing Motherhood: The Mothers of the Plaza de Mayo.* Wilmington, Del.: Scholarly Resources, 1994.

Campbell, D'Ann. *Women at War with America: Private Lives in a Patriotic Era.* Cambridge: Harvard University Press, 1984.

Cannon, Ida M. *On the Social Frontier of Medicine: Pioneering in Medical Social Service.* Cambridge: Harvard University Press, 1952.

Carson, Rachel. *Silent Spring.* Boston: Houghton Mifflin, 1962.

Chandler, Alfred D. *The Visible Hand: The Managerial Revolution in American Business.* Cambridge: Harvard University Press, 1977.

Chavkin, Wendy, ed. *Double Exposure: Women's Health Hazards on the Job and at Home.* New York: Monthly Review Press, 1984.

Cherniak, Martin. *The Hawk's Nest Incident: America's Worst Industrial Disaster.* New Haven: Yale University Press, 1986.

Clark, Claudia. "Glowing in the Dark: The Radium Dial Painters, the Consumers' League and Industrial Health in the United States, 1910–1935." Ph.D. diss., Rutgers University, 1991.

———. "The Menace of Benzene: Alice Hamilton and the Health of American Workers." *Sigerist Circle Newsletter* 8 (Winter 1995).

———. *Radium Girls: Women and Industrial Health Reform, 1910–1935.* Chapel Hill: University of North Carolina Press, 1997.

Cobble, Dorothy Sue. "Recapturing Working-Class Feminism: Union Women in the Postwar Era." In *Not June Cleaver: Women and Gender in Postwar America,* ed. Joanne Meyerowitz, 57–83. Philadelphia: Temple University Press, 1994.

Cohen, Lizabeth. *Making a New Deal: Industrial Workers in Chicago, 1919–1939.* New York: Cambridge University Press, 1990.

Community and Preventive Medicine Department Papers. Medical College of Pennsylvania Archives and Special Collections on Women in Medicine. Philadelphia.

Cook, Blanche Wiesen. *Eleanor Roosevelt,* vol. 1: *1884–1933.* New York: Viking Press, 1992.

Coontz, Stephanie. *The Way We Never Were: American Families and the Nostalgia Trap.* New York: Basic Books, 1992.

Cooper, Jill E. "Keeping the Girls on the Line: The Medical Department and Women Workers at AT&T, 1913–1940." Paper presented at the annual meeting of the American Association for the History of Medicine, Buffalo, New York, May 1996.

Cott, Nancy F. *The Grounding of Modern Feminism.* New Haven: Yale University Press, 1987.

———. "What's in a Name? The Limits of 'Social Feminism'; or Expanding the Vocabulary of Women's History." *Journal of American History* 76 (December 1989): 809–29.

Curran, Jean Alonzo. *Founders: Harvard School of Public Health.* New York: Josiah Macy Foundation, 1970.

Daniels, Cynthia R. *At Women's Expense: State Power and the Politics of Fetal Rights.* Cambridge: Harvard University Press, 1993.

Davies, Marjorie. *Woman's Place Is at the Typewriter: Office Work and Office Workers, 1870–1930.* Philadelphia: Temple University Press, 1982.

Davis, Allen F. *American Heroine: The Life and Legend of Jane Addams.* London: Oxford University Press, 1973.

———. *Spearheads for Reform: The Social Settlements and the Progressive Movement, 1890–1914.* New York: Oxford University Press, 1967.

Degler, Carl. *In Search of Human Nature: The Decline and Revival of Darwinism in American Social Thought.* Oxford: Oxford University Press, 1991.

Derickson, Alan. "Physiological Science and Scientific Management in the Progressive Era: Frederic S. Lee and the Committee on Industrial Fatigue." *Business History Review* 68 (Winter 1994): 484–513.

———. *Workers' Health, Workers' Democracy: The Western Miners' Struggle, 1891–1925.* Ithaca: Cornell University Press, 1988.

Doyal, Leslie. *What Makes Women Sick: Gender and the Political Economy of Health.* New Brunswick: Rutgers University Press, 1995.

Duffy, John. *A History of Public Health in New York City,* 2 vols. New York: Russell Sage Foundation, 1968, 1974.

———. "Social Impact of Disease in the Late Nineteenth Century." In *Sickness and Health in America: Readings in the History of Medicine and Public Health.* 2d rev. ed., ed. Judith Walzer Leavitt and Ronald L. Numbers, 414–21. Madison: University of Wisconsin Press, 1985.

Erickson, Nancy. "*Muller v. Oregon* Reconsidered: The Origins of a Sex-Based Doctrine of Liberty of Contract." *Labor History* 30 (1989): 228–50.

Evans, Sara. *Born for Liberty: A History of Women in America.* New York: Free Press, 1989.

Fitzpatrick, Ellen. *Endless Crusade: Women Social Scientists and Progressive Reform.* Oxford: Oxford University Press, 1990.

Flanagan, Maureen. "Gender and Urban Political Reform: The City Club and the Women's City Club of Chicago in the Progressive Era." *American Historical Review* 95 (October 1995): 1032–51.

Fox, Steve. *Toxic Work: Women Workers at GTE Lenkurt.* Philadelphia: Temple University Press, 1991.

Gabin, Nancy F. *Feminism in the Labor Movement: Women and the United Auto Workers, 1935–1975.* Ithaca: Cornell University Press, 1990.

Galishoff, Stuart. *Safeguarding the Public Health: Newark, 1895–1918.* Westport, Conn.: Greenwood Press, 1975.

Gersuny, Carl. *Work Hazards and Industrial Conflict.* Hanover, N.H.: University Press of New England, 1981.

Gillespie, Richard. *Manufacturing Knowledge: A History of the Hawthorne Experiments.* Cambridge: Cambridge University Press, 1991.

Glazer, Penina, and Miriam Slater. *Unequal Colleagues: The Entrance of Women into the Professions, 1890–1940.* New Brunswick: Rutgers University Press, 1987.

Gluck, Sherna Berger. *Rosie the Riveter Revisited: Women, the War, and Social Change.* Boston: Twayne, 1989.

Golden, Janet. "Creating FAS, or: Doctors Can Discover Disease but It Takes a Whole Society to Make a Syndrome." Paper presented at the annual meeting of the American Association for the History of Medicine, Buffalo, New York, May 1996.

———. "Trouble in the Nursery: Physicians, Families and Wet Nurses at the End of the Nineteenth Century." In *"To Toil the Livelong Day": America's Women at Work, 1780–1980,* ed. Carol Groneman and Mary Beth Norton, 125–37. Ithaca: Cornell University Press, 1987.

Goldin, Claudia. *Understanding the Gender Gap: An Economic History of American Women.* Philadelphia: University of Pennsylvania Press, 1991.

Goldmark, Josephine. *Fatigue and Efficiency: A Study in Industry.* New York: Russell Sage Foundation, 1912.

Gordon, Linda. *Heroes of Their Own Lives: The Politics and History of Family Violence, Boston, 1880–1960.* New York: Penguin Books, 1988.

———. "The New Feminist Scholarship on the Welfare State," In *Women, the State, and Welfare,* ed. Linda Gordon, 9–35. Madison: University of Wisconsin Press, 1990.

———. *Pitied but Not Entitled: Single Mothers and the History of Welfare, 1890–1935.* Cambridge: Harvard University Press, 1994.

———. *Woman's Body, Woman's Right: A Social History of Birth Control in America.* New York: Viking Press, 1976.

Gould, Stephen Jay. *The Mismeasure of Man.* New York: W. W. Norton, 1981.

Jean Gowing Papers. Medical College of Pennsylvania Archives and Special Collections on Women in Medicine. Philadelphia.

Greenwald, Maurine W. *Women, War, and Work: The Impact of World War I on Women Workers in the United States.* Westport, Conn.: Greenwood Press, 1980.

Hamilton, Alice. *Exploring the Dangerous Trades: The Autobiography of Alice Hamilton.* Boston: Little, Brown, 1943.

Hardy, Harriet L. *Challenging Man-Made Disease: The Memoirs of Harriet L. Hardy, M.D.* New York: Praeger, 1983.

Hartmann, Susan. *The Home Front and Beyond: American Women in the 1940s.* Boston: Twayne, 1982.

Hays, Samuel P., and Barbara D. Hays. *Beauty, Health, and Permanence: Environmental Politics in the United States, 1955–1985.* Cambridge: Cambridge University Press, 1987.

Heifetz, Ruth. "Women, Lead, and Reproductive Hazards: Defining a New Risk." In *Dying for Work: Workers' Safety and Health in Twentieth-Century America,* ed. David Rosner and Gerald Markowitz, 160–75. Bloomington: Indiana University Press, 1989.

Hendricks, Rickey. *A Model for National Health Care: The History of Kaiser Permanente.* New Brunswick: Rutgers University Press, 1993.

Herber, Lewis. *Our Synthetic Environment.* New York: Alfred A. Knopf, 1962.

Hill, Ann Corinne. "Protection of Women Workers and the Courts: A Legal Case History." *Feminist Studies* 5 (Summer 1979): 247–73.

Hill, Patricia Evridge. "Redefining Occupational Illness: Mill Work, Maternal Health, Social Class and Women's Roles in the Textile South." *Sigerist Circle Newsletter* 8 (Winter 1995): 3–5.

Hospital of the University of Pennsylvania Papers. University of Pennsylvania Archives. Philadelphia.

Hossfeld, Karen. "'Their Logic Against Them': Contradictions in Sex, Race, and Class in Silicon Valley." In *Women Workers in Global Restructuring,* ed. Kathryn Ward, 149–78. Ithaca, N.Y.: ILR Press, 1990.

Hough, Mazie. "'I'm a Poor Girl in Family and I Want to Know If You Be Kind': The Community's Response to Unwed Mothers in Maine and Tennessee, 1876–1954." Ph.D. diss., University of Maine, 1997.

Howell, Joel. *Technology in the Hospital: Transforming Patient Care in the Early Twentieth Century.* Baltimore: Johns Hopkins University Press, 1995.

Hunt, Vilma. *Work and the Health of Women.* Boca Raton, Fla.: CRC Press, 1979.

———. "A Brief History of Women Workers and Hazards in the Workplace." *Feminist Studies* 5 (Summer 1979): 274–85.

International Union of Electrical Workers Papers. Rutgers University Libraries. New Brunswick, New Jersey.

Kenney, Sally J. *For Whose Protection? Reproductive Hazards and Exclusionary Policies in the United States and Great Britain.* Ann Arbor: University of Michigan Press, 1992.

Kessler-Harris, Alice. *Out to Work: A History of Wage-Earning Women in the United States.* Oxford: Oxford University Press, 1982.

———. "The Paradox of Motherhood: Night Work Restrictions in the United States." In *Protecting Women: Labor Legislation in Europe, the United States, and Australia, 1880–1920,* ed. Ulla Wikander, Alice Kessler-Harris, and Jane Lewis, 337–57. Urbana: University of Illinois Press, 1995.

———. "Problems of Coalition-Building: Women and the Trade Unions in the 1920s." In *Women, Work, and Protest: A Century of U.S. Women's Labor History,* ed. Ruth Milkman, 110–38. New York: Routledge Press, 1985.

Klein, Patricia Vawter. "'For the Good of the Race': Reproductive Hazards from Lead and the Persistence of Exclusionary Policies toward Women." In *Women, Work, and Technology: Transformations,* ed. Barbara Drygulski et al. Ann Arbor: University of Michigan Press, 1987.

Kotelchuck, David. "Asbestos: 'The Funeral Dress of Kings'—and Others." In *Dying for Work: Workers' Safety and Health in Twentieth-Century America,* ed. David Rosner and Gerald Markowitz, 192–207. Bloomington: Indiana University Press, 1989.

Kunzel, Regina. *Fallen Women, Problem Girls: Unmarried Mothers and the Professionalization of Social Work, 1890–1945.* New Haven: Yale University Press, 1993.

Leavitt, Judith Walzer. *The Healthiest City: Milwaukee and the Politics of Health Reform.* Princeton: Princeton University Press, 1982.

Lehrer, Susan. *Origins of Protective Labor Legislation for Women, 1905–1925.* Albany: State University of New York Press, 1987.

Luker, Kristen. *Abortion and the Politics of Motherhood.* Berkeley: University of California Press, 1984.

Malone, Carolyn. "Gender, Work and the State: Government Regulation of Women's Work in the White Lead Trades in England, 1891–1898." Paper presented at the annual North American Labor History Conference, Detroit, Michigan, November 1994.

Marsh, Margaret, and Wanda Ronner. *The Empty Cradle: Infertility in America from Colonial Times to the Present.* Baltimore: Johns Hopkins University Press, 1996.

Martin, Emily. *The Woman in the Body: A Cultural Analysis of Reproduction.* Boston: Beacon Press, 1992.

Mass, William, and Charles Levenstein. "Labor Relations, Technology, and Occupational Disease: Banning the Suck Shuttle in Massachusetts, 1911." Paper presented at the Business History Conference, Hartford, Connecticut, March 1984.

McGaw, Judith A. *Most Wonderful Machine: Mechanization and Social Change in Berkshire Paper Making, 1801–1843.* Princeton: Princeton University Press, 1987.

Mead, Rebecca. "Eggs for Sale." *New Yorker.* August 9, 1999.

Meckel, Richard A. *Save the Babies: American Public Health Reform and the Prevention of Infant Mortality, 1850–1929.* Baltimore: Johns Hopkins University Press, 1990.

Medical College of Pennsylvania Public Relations Department Papers. Medical College of Pennsylvania Archives and Special Collections on Women in Medicine. Philadelphia.

Merchant, Carolyn. *Ecological Revolutions: Nature, Gender, and Science in New England.* Chapel Hill: University of North Carolina Press, 1989.

Milkman, Ruth. "Redefining 'Women's Work': The Sexual Division of Labor in the Auto Industry during World War II." In *Women and Power in American History: A Reader,* vol. 2: *Since 1870,* ed. Kathryn Kish Sklar and Thomas Dublin, 209–22. Englewood Cliffs, N.J.: Prentice-Hall, 1991.

———. "Women's History and the Sears Case." *Feminist Studies* 12 (1986): 375–400.

Morantz-Sanchez, Regina Markell. *Sympathy and Science: Women Physicians in American Medicine.* New York: Oxford University Press, 1985.

Mosely, George. "Our Babies, Ourselves: What Some Call Protecting the Unborn, Others, Including the Supreme Court, Call Sex Discrimination." *Business and Health* 9 (June 1991).

Muncy, Robyn. *Creating a Female Dominion in American Reform.* Oxford: Oxford University Press, 1991.

Nathan, Maud. *The Story of an Epoch-Making Movement.* New York: Doubleday, 1926.

New York State Factory Investigating Commission. New York State Archives and Records Administration. Albany.

Noble, Charles. *Liberalism at Work: The Rise and Fall of OSHA.* Philadelphia: Temple University Press, 1986.

Nugent, Angela. "The Power to Define a New Disease: Epidemiological Politics and Radium Poisoning." In *Dying for Work: Workers' Safety and Health in Twentieth-Century America,* ed. David Rosner and Gerald Markowitz, 179–91. Bloomington: University of Indiana Press, 1989.

Offen, Karen. "Deciding Feminism: A Comparative Historical Approach." *Signs* 14 (Autumn 1988): 119–57.

Office of Technology Assessment. *Reproductive Health Hazards in the Workplace.* Washington: Government Printing Office, 1985.

Page, Joseph A., and Mary-Win O'Brien. *Bitter Wages: Ralph Nader's Study Group Report on Disease and Injury on the Job.* New York: Grossman, 1973.

Parlee, Mary Brown. "Contestation and Consolidation in Scientific Discourses about Premenstrual Syndrome." Paper presented at the Ninth Berkshire Conference on the History of Women, Vassar College, June 11, 1993.

Petchesky, Rosalind. "Workers, Reproductive Hazards and the Politics of Protection: An Introduction." *Feminist Studies* 5 (Summer 1979): 233–46.

Phelps, Elizabeth Stuart. *The Silent Partner.* 1871. Reprint, New York: Feminist Press, 1983.

Pleck, Elizabeth. *Domestic Tyranny: The Making of Social Policy against Family Violence from Colonial Times to the Present.* Oxford: Oxford University Press, 1987.

Polenberg, Richard. *War and Society: The United States, 1941–1945.* Philadelphia: J. B. Lippincott, 1972.

Reed, James. *The Birth Control Movement and American Society: From Private Vice to Public Virtue.* Princeton: Princeton University Press, 1978.

Reeve, Patricia. "Injured in the Service of the Commonwealth: Massachusetts Industrial Soldiers Seek Recompense, 1881–1887." Paper presented at the annual meeting of the New England Historical Association, Mount Holyoke College, South Hadley, Massachusetts, April 29, 1995.

Reiser, Stanley Joel. *Medicine and the Reign of Technology.* Cambridge: Cambridge University Press, 1978.

Robinson, James C., and Mita Giacomini. "A Reallocation of Rights in Industries with Reproductive Health Hazards." *Milbank Quarterly* 70 (Winter 1992): 587–604.

Rogers, Naomi. *Dirt and Disease: Polio before FDR.* New Brunswick: Rutgers University Press, 1992.

Rosenberg, Charles E. "The Bitter Fruit: Heredity, Disease and Social Thought." In *No Other Gods: On Science and American Social Thought,* ed. Charles E. Rosenberg, 25–53. Baltimore: Johns Hopkins University Press, 1976.

———. *The Cholera Years: The United States in 1832, 1849, and 1866.* 1962. Reprint, Chicago: University of Chicago Press, 1987.

———. "The Therapeutic Revolution: Medicine, Meaning, and Social Change in Nineteenth-Century America." In *The Therapeutic Revolution: Essays in the Social History of Medicine,* ed. Morris J. Vogel and Charles E. Rosenberg, 3–25. Philadelphia: University of Pennsylvania Press, 1979.

Rosenkrantz, Barbara Gutmann. *Public Health and the State: Changing Views in Massachusetts, 1842–1936.* Cambridge: Harvard University Press, 1972.

Rosner, David, and Gerald Markowitz. *Deadly Dust: Silicosis and the Politics of Occupational Disease in Twentieth-Century America.* Princeton: Princeton University Press, 1991.

———. "The Early Movement for Occupational Safety and Health, 1900–1917." In *Sickness and Health in America: Readings in the History of Medicine and Public Health*, 2d rev. ed., ed. Judith Walzer Leavitt and Ronald L. Numbers, 507–21. Madison: University of Wisconsin Press, 1985.

———. "'A Gift of God'?: The Public Health Controversy over Leaded Gasoline during the 1920s." In *Dying for Work: Workers' Safety and Health in Twentieth-Century America*, ed. David Rosner and Gerald Markowitz, 121–39. Bloomington: Indiana University Press, 1989.

———. "Research or Advocacy: Federal Occupational Safety and Health Policies during the New Deal." In *Dying for Work: Workers' Safety and Health in Twentieth-Century America*, ed. David Rosner and Gerald Markowitz, 83–102. Bloomington: Indiana University Press, 1989.

Rupp, Leila, and Verta Taylor. *Survival in the Doldrums: The American Women's Rights Movement, 1945 to the 1960s.* Oxford: Oxford University Press, 1987.

Russell Sage Foundation Papers. Rockefeller Archives Center, Tarrytown, New York.

Russett, Cynthia Eagle. *Sexual Science: The Victorian Construction of Womanhood.* Cambridge: Harvard University Press, 1989.

Ryan, Mary. *Womanhood in America: From Colonial Times to the Present.* 3d ed. New York: Franklin Watts, 1983.

Sapiro, Virgina, ed. *Women, Biology and Public Policy.* Beverly Hills, Calif.: Sage Publications, 1985.

Sarvasy, Wendy. "Beyond the Difference versus Equality Debate: Postsuffrage Feminism, Citizenship, and the Quest for a Feminist Welfare State." *Signs* 17 (Winter 1992): 329–62.

Scott, Joan. "Gender as a Useful Category of Analysis." *American Historical Review* 91 (October 1985): 1053–75.

Scott, Judith. "Keeping Women in Their Place: Exclusionary Policies and Reproduction." In *Double Exposure: Women's Health Hazards on the Job and at Home*, ed. Wendy Chavkin, 180–95. New York: Monthly Review Press, 1984.

Sellers, Christopher. "The Public Health Service's Office of Industrial Hygiene and the Transformation of Industrial Medicine." *Bulletin of the History of Medicine* 65 (Spring 1991): 42–73.

———. *Hazards of the Job: From Industrial Disease to Environmental Health Science.* Chapel Hill: University of North Carolina Press, 1997.

Shilts, Randy. *And the Band Played On: Politics, People, and the AIDS Epidemic.* New York: Viking Press, 1987.

Shorter, Edward. *From Paralysis to Fatigue: A History of Psychosomatic Illness in the Modern Era.* New York: Free Press, 1992.

Sicherman, Barbara. *Alice Hamilton: A Life in Letters.* Cambridge: Harvard University Press, 1984.

———. "Working It Out: Gender, Profession and Reform in the Career of Alice Hamilton." In *Gender, Class, Race, and Reform in the Progressive Era*, ed. Noralee Frankel and Nancy Schrom Dye, 127–47. Lexington: University of Kentucky Press, 1991.

Sklar, Kathryn Kish. *Florence Kelley and the Nation's Work.* New Haven: Yale University Press, 1995.

———. "Why Were Most Politically Active Women Opposed to the ERA in the 1920s?" In *Women and Power in American History: A Reader,* vol. 2: *From 1870,* ed. Kathryn Kish Sklar and Thomas Dublin, 175–82. Englewood Cliffs, N.J.: Prentice-Hall, 1991.

Skocpol, Theda. *Protecting Soldiers and Mothers: The Political Origins of Social Policy in the United States.* Cambridge: Harvard University Press, 1992.

Smith, Barbara Ellen. *Digging Our Own Graves: Coal Miners and the Struggle over Black Lung.* Philadelphia: Temple University Press, 1987.

Smith-Rosenberg, Carroll. *Disorderly Conduct: Visions of Gender in Victorian America.* Oxford: Oxford University Press, 1985.

Snyder, Lynne Page. "'The Death-Dealing Smog over Donora, Pennsylvania': Industrial Air Pollution, Public Health, and Federal Policy, 1915–1963." Ph.D. diss., University of Pennsylvania, 1994.

Starr, Paul. *The Social Transformation of American Medicine: The Rise of a Sovereign Profession and the Making of a Vast Industry.* New York: Basic Books, 1982.

Stellman, Jeanne Mager. *Women's Work, Women's Health: Myths and Realities.* New York: Pantheon Books, 1977.

Stellman, Jeanne Mager, and Susan M. Daum. *Work Is Dangerous to Your Health.* New York: Random House, 1973.

Stevens, Rosemary. *American Medicine and the Public Interest.* New Haven: Yale University Press, 1971.

Tuttle, William M. *Daddy's Gone to War: The Second World War in the Lives of America's Children.* Oxford: Oxford University Press, 1993.

Uterine Cancer Cytology Research Project. Medical College of Pennsylvania Archives and Special Collections on Women in Medicine. Philadelphia.

Vogel, Lise. *Mothers on the Job: Maternity Policy in the U.S. Workplace.* New Brunswick: Rutgers University Press, 1993.

Vogel, Morris J. *The Invention of the Modern Hospital: Boston, 1870–1930.* Chicago: University of Chicago Press, 1980.

White, Richard. "Environmental History, Ecology and Meaning." *Journal of American History* 76 (March 1990): 1111–6.

Whorton, James. *Before Silent Spring: Pesticides and Public Health in Pre-DDT America.* Princeton: Princeton University Press, 1974.

Wiebe, Robert H. *The Search for Order, 1877–1920.* New York: Hill and Wang, 1967.

Woloch, Nancy. *Muller v. Oregon: A Brief History with Documents.* New York: St. Martin's Press, 1996.

Women and Environmental History. Special issue of *Environmental Review* 8 (Spring 1984).

Worster, Donald. *The Wealth of Nature: Environmental History and the Ecological Imagination.* New York: Oxford University Press, 1993.

Wright, Michael. "Reproductive Hazards and 'Protective' Discrimination." *Feminist Studies* 5 (Summer 1979): 302–9.

Young, James Harvey. "Patent Medicines and the Self-Help Syndrome." In *Sickness and Health in America: Readings in the History of Medicine and Public Health*. 2d rev. ed., ed. Judith Walzer Leavitt and Ronald L. Numbers, 71–8. Madison: University of Wisconsin Press, 1985.

Index

Absenteeism, of women during World War II, 8, 79–81
Age, risk factor in industrial disease, 98
Aircraft industry, employment of women during World War II, 68
American Academy for the Advancement of Science, 123
American Cyanamid Corp., fetal protection policy, 124
Archives of Environmental Health, 111
Asbestos, workplace health: during World War II, 74; after World War II, 119
Automobile industry, employment of women during World War II, 74; and lead, 119

Baetjer, Dr. Anna, on lead poisoning and effect on fetuses, 115
Barney, Nora Stanton, 104
Benzene: health effects, 33, 39, 41, 100; industrial uses, 40, 41, 42
Benzene poisoning, 39, 77; and Alice Hamilton, 93; Consumers' League of Massachusetts, 40
Biological differences, effect on ERA, 90, 91
Boston Chamber of Commerce, 1910 survey, 16, 17
Boycotts, as strategy of Consumers' Leagues, 50
Brandeis, Louis, and *Muller v. Oregon*, 23

Bureaucrats, as former reformers, 47, 53
Business owners, response to industrial health and industrial life, 16, 18. *See also* Industrial welfare

Cabot, Dr. Richard C., and medical social services at Massachusetts General Hospital, 21
Calcium, effects of lead poisoning on, 115
Campbell, James (Pennsylvania factory inspector), 14
Candy factories, 48, 94
Can manufacturing, benzene use, 41
Cannon, Ida: medical social work and industrial health, 21; single motherhood, 117
Carson, Rachel, and environmental health, 111
Carter's Ink, and workplace health, 17
Chemical hazards, increased risk during World War II, 70
Children, effect of mother's workplace conditions on, 15, 16
Consumerism, and workers' health, 50, 112
Consumers' League, New York City: department store clerks, 47, 48; industrial homework, 48; "White List," 49
Consumers' League, Ohio, and women grinders, 99
Consumers' League of Massachusetts, benzene poisoning, 40

171

Consumers' League of New Jersey: "powder puffs," 48; radiation poisoning, 108; radium dial painting, 42
Consumers' Leagues, and working women's health, 39, 50
Council on Occupational Health (AMA), support for working women in 1961, 120
Counselors, woman: employment of during World War II, 80, 81

Departments of labor, state: responsibility for workplace conditions, 35
Department stores: industrial welfare programs, 18; and women's health, 47
Dermatitis, in industry, 65
Dickens, Charles, description of lead poisoning in *The Uncommercial Traveler,* 32
Domestic service, and protective labor legislation, 4
Double duty, 2, 118, 120, 128; cause of absenteeism, 79, 80, 81; and Alice Hamilton, 85; in World War II, 67, 79
DuPont Corp., fetal protection policy, 124
Dysmenorrhea, 60, 78

Efficiency: influence of Frederick Winslow Taylor, 25; relationship between home and workplace, 61
Emphysema, detected in pre-employment physical exams, 70
Environment: household, 107; human health, 12, 13, 81; neighborhood, 18; workplace, 93
Environmental hazards, 8, 112; polyvinyl chloride, 110; radiation, 108
Environmental health, 109–10
Environmental history, 4

Environmentalism: community hazards, 111, 113; and gender, 4, 26; and modern medicine, 20, 22, 26; workplace, 51, 61, 102, 108; workplace health, 35, 57, 62
Equal Employment Opportunity Commission, conflict over state protective labor legislation, 122
Equality, in workplace, 81, 82
Equal Rights Amendment (ERA): feminism, 52, 86, 90, 91; and individualism, 86; opposition to, 51, 52, 86, 100; sources of support, 8, 70, 83, 87; and Women's Bureau, 55; workplace, 2, 7; workplace health, 5, 55, 78, 89
Equal Rights feminism, and women workers, 52
Exxon Corp., fetal protection policy, 124

Factory inspections: discovery of workplace hazards, 34; gender-specific concerns, 14; New Jersey, 14; as "opening wedge," 14; Pennsylvania, 11, 14
Fatigue: and double duty, 80; and "Hawthorne Effect," 64; relationship to industrial health, 24, 25, 65; research during World War II, 79; and Frederick Winslow Taylor, 25
Fatigue and Efficiency (Goldmark): dangers to women, 24–25; telephone operators, 49–50
Femininity, 71
Feminism: definitions, 5, 52; effect on women's workplace health, 5, 86, 91, 113; individualism, 92; and personal responsibility, 113; relationship to modern medicine, 92; significance of biological differences, 113; and welfare state, 90
Fertility, effects of lead poisoning on, 115

Fetal protection policies, 8, 114, 115–18, 124; American Cyanamid, 124; economic concerns, 116, 128; feminist debate over, 114, 117, 123; impact on work opportunities for women, 119, 123; General Motors foundries, 114; Johnson Controls, 124

Fetal rights, impact on workplace, 9

Filth theory, 12, 13

Foundries, women's exclusion from, 38, 88, 104

Frankford Arsenal, 73

Garment manufacturing, performed at home, 48

Gender: family and community, 15; and workplace health, 1, 9

Germ theory, 12

Gilbreth, Lillian, 106

Goldmark, Josephine, application of scientific tests on fatigue, 24; and *Muller v. Oregon*, 23. See also *Fatigue and Efficiency*

Grinding and polishing, 99, 104

Gynecology, treatment of infertility, 30

H.J. Heinz Corp., 17

Hair spray, risks to beauticians and consumers, 119, 120

Hair, and women's safety during World War II, 72, 73

Hamilton, Dr. Alice: attitude toward industrial physicians, 57; benzene, 39, 41; environmentalism and health, 93; and ERA, 6, 83, 99, 100; feminism, 6, 23, 37, 83, 85, 95; gender and health, 91, 94, 95; hatting industry in 1924, 66; industrial hazards, 28, 66, 98; and Florence Kitchelt, 99; lead 28, 37, 38; Elizabeth Magee, 100; medical influences, 83, 93; Medical Women's National Association in 1924, 87; National Consumers' League, leadership in, 83, 98; poverty, 37, 92; protective labor legislation, 5, 23, 37, 84, 85, 94, 96, 99; public health, 96; radium dial painters, 95; reformist influences, 83, 96; support for UN Commission on Human Rights, 99; working women, 28, 92, 94

Hardy, Dr. Harriet L., 109

Hatting industry, 66

Hawes, Elizabeth (*New York Times* writer), 67

Hawthorne Effect, 64

Hazardous materials, women's exposure during World War II, 74

Health, relationship to environment, 13

Hemorrhage, associated with benzene, 33

Higher education, effect on reproductive capacity of women, 29

Housework: "pathology and hygiene of housework" conference in 1950, 105–8

Hricko, Andrea, 123

Hull House, effect on Hamilton's work, 96

Hunt, Dr. Vilma, 123

Industrial chemicals, hazardous, control of, 31, 33, 34

Industrial Clinic, Massachusetts General Hospital, 20, 22

Industrial disease, 60, 116

Industrial hazards, during World War II, 97

Industrial health, 11; and fatigue, 24; relationship to occupational health, 109

Industrial homework, 48

Industrial hygiene: Europe compared to United States, 31; relationship between home and workplace, 46, 47, 61, 62

Industrial hygienists, 58

Industrial medicine, 34, 103, 112
Industrial physicians, 56, 57, 58, 102; Alice Hamilton's disappointment with, 57; relationship between workplace and personal life, 102
Industrial welfare, 17, 18, 19; during World War II, 80; relationship to occupational health, 17; use of industrial nurses, 17
Industrial workplace, in comparison to housework, 108
Infant mortality, and public health, 30
Infertility, treatment of women, 30
International efforts, employment discrimination and workplace health, 124
International Union of Electrical Workers, and fetal protection policies, 118
Ionizing radiation, and workplace health after World War II, 119

Jacobi, Dr. Mary Putnam, working women's and children's health, 15
Johnson Controls: impact on local economy, 6; suit against fetal protection policy, 124

Kehoe, Robert, 59
Kellogg, Paul, 65
Kitchelt, Florence, 99

Ladies' Home Journal, article by Alice Hamilton, 98
Lakeman, Mary, dysmenorrhea study, 60
Laundries, reproductive risks to women, 38
Lead: American Public Health Association standards, 42; in industry, 31, 33, 38, 43, 76, 119; and personal hygiene, 39; regulation, 35, 37, 118; risks to women, 35, 36, 38; risks to workers, 37, 39, 118; after World War II, 119

Lead poisoning: in children, 46; description of by Charles Dickens, 32; diagnosis, 33, 58, 60; effects on women, 28, 42, 43, 95, 115; in industry, 32, 38, 57, 76; and Robert Kehoe, 59; and May Mayers, 59; and National Lead Company, 57; protection of women from, 76, 77, 95
Lead poisoning, chronic, 32, 114; diagnosis, 59; effect on reproduction, 114
Lifting hazards, during World War II, 73

Magee, Elizabeth, correspondence with Hamilton on ERA, 99, 100
Manufacturers' Research Association, industrial health and safety, 62, 63
Marinship Company, 73
Maternal health, relationship to modern medicine, 7, 45, 94
Maximum weight laws, effect on working women, 73, 74
Mayers, May, 59, 60
Mayo, Elton, and fatigue, 64
Medical services, industrial, effect on occupational health, 62
Medical social service department, Massachusetts General Hospital, 21
Medical social workers, and industrial health, 21
Medical Women's International Association (MWIA), international study of housework, 105, 106
Medical Women's National Association, and ERA, 87, 88
Medicine, modern, 12, 20; feminism and, 89, 92; gender, 8; workplace health, 8, 20, 27
Menstruation, 61
Metal Wire Recovery Company, use of polyvinyl chloride, 110
Minimum wage legislation, and women's health, 53, 54
Miscarriages, effects of lead, 36

Motherhood: changing definitions, 3, 14, 30, 114, 128; health, 3, 30, 114; and positions on ERA, 85; reproductive technology, 129

Muller v. Oregon, support for protective labor legislation, 23

Munitions industry, employment of women during World War II, 68

National Consumers' League: and benzene, 40; and radiation hazards, 109

National Lead Company, and lead poisoning, 57

National Safety Council, 72

National Woman's Party, 63, 76, 97; and male reproductive health, 118; during World War II, 78

Neo-Lamarckianism, 16

Niagara Falls, industrial lead poisoning during World War I, 38

Nightwork: and effect on World War II, 70; *Radice v. The People of the State of New York,* 53; and women's health, 15

Nurses, industrial, use in industrial welfare programs, 17

O'Brien, Dr. Thomas, warning about lead poisoning, 46

Occupational disease, 35, 44, 47; individual approach to health, 44; non-gendered aspects of, 36; non-occupational causes of, 58

Occupational health, 1, 12, 17, 20, 99, 103, 109; and gender, 67, 68, 92; and World War II, 67, 102

Oil, Chemical and Atomic Workers Union, and fetal protection policies, 118

Oliver, Dr. Thomas: influence on Pennsylvania regulations, 38; on risks of lead to women, 36

Operating room personnel, workplace hazards, 123

Our Bodies, Ourselves, 121

"Pathology and hygiene of housework" session, 1950 MWIA conference, 105

Pelvic exams, use of in pre-employment physical exams, 76

Perkins, Frances: on falling accidents, 72; New York State Department of Labor, 53; position on ERA, 89

Phelps, Elizabeth Stuart, description of workers in *The Silent Partner,* 13

Phosphorus, industrial use of, 33

Physical defects, and pre-employment physical exams, 70

Polyvinyl chloride, industrial hazards of, 110

Poverty, and workplace health, 37, 54, 55, 93, 94

Powder puffs, industrial homework manufacturing, 48

Pre-employment physical exams, 63, 70, 71, 102

Pregnancy: effect of working conditions on, 75, 94; employment standards regarding, 75, 122; feminist debate over in 1975, 123; and lead poisoning, 115; medical evidence regarding risks at work, 75

Pregnancy Discrimination Act, 123

Pre-placement physical exams, 63

Printers, women, and nightwork, 23

Protection, definitions of, 88

Protectionism, 7, 92, 120

Protective labor legislation, 22, 24; and biological differences, 91; impact of Civil Rights Act of 1964, 121, 122; and class, 6, 50; economic effects, 4, 64; as "entering wedge," 97; feminist support for, 86; and fetal protection policies, 114; gender, 4, 50, 86, 91;

Protective labor legislation (*continued*) and Alice Hamilton, 84, 85, 94, 98; institutionalization of, 53, 97; legitimacy, 8, 70, 74, 81, 82, 86, 104; *Muller v. Oregon,* 23; and National Woman's Party, 97; *Radice v. The People of the State of New York,* 53; rationale, 12, 22, 23, 53, 70, 87, 97; relationship to environmentalism, 2, 12; relationship to medicine, 24, 89, 91, 96; selectivity, 4, 23, 55, 89; state regulations, 23, 24; and United Auto Workers, 118

Public health: environmentalism, 20; new, 57; working-class maternal and child health, 30, 78, 96

Radice v. The People of the State of New York, 53
Radium dial painters, occupational disease, 95
Radium poisoning, 42, 58
Reformers, 16, 47; industrial welfare, 19; workplace health, 7
Reproduction, scientific attention to, 29, 30
Reproductive hazards, 16, 28, 85, 121
Reproductive health, use in employment decisions, 120, 121
Reproductive technology, 129

Shipbuilding industry, employment of women during World War II, 68, 76
Silent Spring (Carson), effect on occupational health professionals, 111
Silica, and workplace health after World War II, 119
Smelting plant workers, working and living conditions, 93
Specialization: and environmentalism, 22; industrial medicine, 20; in society, 19

Spray enameling industry, risks of lead poisoning, 42
Stellman, Jeanne Mager, 123
Stevens, Doris, 92
Stillbirths, effects of lead, 36
Storage battery manufacturing, 93
Sturgis, Dr. Katharine, 103; Metal Wire Recovery study, 110–11
Suck shuttle, in textile factories, 26
Survey, Hamilton's article on hatting industry, 66
Synovitis, in industry, 65

Taylor, Frederick Winslow, efficiency studies in industry, 25
Telephone operators, and efficiency, 49, 50
Tetra-ethyl lead, acute poisoning of oil workers in 1924, 58
Textile mills: manufacturers' criticism of state protective labor laws, 64; suck shuttle, 26; working conditions, 13, 26, 87
Textile workers, description of in Phelps's *The Silent Partner,* 13
Thesaurosis (pulmonary disease from hair spray), 119
Tobacco processing, reproductive risks to women, 38
Tuberculosis, incidence in textile factories, 26

United Auto Workers, response to fetal protection policies, 118
United States Radium Corporation, and radium poisoning, 95
Urbanization, rationale for social reform, 19
Uterine Cancer Cytology Research project, 103

Van Kleeck, Mary: opposition to ERA, 88; and women's health, 15

War Manpower Commission, 68, 71
Wartime industries, employment of women in, 68. *See also specific industries*
Watchorn, Robert (Pennsylvania factory inspector), 11
"Welder's wheeze," 75
Welding hazards, in shipyards and aircraft plants, 75
"White List," in New York City, 49
Women's Bureau: advocacy for working women, 54, 55, 65; ERA, 55, 76, 100; protective labor legislation, 55, 64, 75, 76, 97; research, 54, 65, 68, 75, 77, 79; impact of World War II, 68, 75, 76, 77, 97, 104, 105
Women's bureaus, state and federal, promotion of working women's health, 53
Women's Joint Congressional Committee, opposition to ERA, 87
Women's Trade Union League, and working women's health, 14
Women welders, 71, 74
Women workers: and domestic responsibilities, 67; economic disadvantages of, 92; environmentalism, 26; equality of risk, 113; fatigue, 25; femininity and stereotypes, 71, 72, 73; implications of feminism, 9, 67, 91; regulations, 73, 87, 88, 120; as research subjects, 22, 60; textile mills, 87; working conditions, 25, 71, 73, 79, 93, 113. *See also* Double duty; Protective labor legislation
Workers: health and hiring, 63, 103, 121; and occupational health professionals, 112; responsibility for ill health, 19, 45, 47; subjects for medical studies, 111
Workers' compensation, 69, 115, 119; gynecological and obstetrical problems, 116
Working conditions: housework, 106; and modern consumerism, 50; poverty, 93; World War II, 68
Working women. *See* Women workers
Workplace, household as, 107
Workplace changes, accommodation to women's differences, 74
Workplace conditions, women's social identity, 2, 13
Workplace discrimination, international perspectives, 127
Workplace environment: effect of fetal protection policies, 117, 128; gender, 127, 128
Workplace hazards, 34; gynecological and obstetrical problems, 116; operating room personnel, 123; in predominantly female industries, 105; during World War II, 70
Workplace health: in candy factories, 94; ERA, 5; and hiring, 63, 121; international context, 127; Neo-Lamarckianism, influences of, 16; personal responsibility for, 2, 63, 102; and poverty, 37, 94; and pregnancy, 94; relationship to environment, 35, 93; relationship to medicine, 3, 13; and woman counselors, 81
World War I, effects on women workers, 36
World War II, 8, 67–82, 102

Women and Health Series
Cultural and Social Perspectives

Rima D. Apple and Janet Golden, Editors

The series examines the social and cultural construction of health practices and policies, focusing on women as subjects and objects of medical theory, health services, and policy formulation.

Mothers and Motherhood
Readings in American History
Edited by Rima D. Apple and Janet Golden

Modern Mothers in the Heartland
Gender, Health, and Progress in Illinois, 1900–1930
Lynne Curry

Making Midwives Legal
Childbirth, Medicine, and the Law, second edition
Raymond G. DeVries

Travels with the Wolf
A Story of Chronic Illness
Melissa Anne Goldstein

The Selling of Contraception
The Dalkon Shield Case, Sexuality, and Women's Autonomy
Nicole J. Grant

Crack Mothers
Pregnancy, Drugs, and the Media
Drew Humphries

And Sin No More
Social Policy and Unwed Mothers in Cleveland, 1855–1990
Marian J. Morton

Women and Prenatal Testing
Facing the Challenges of Genetic Technology
Edited by Karen H. Rothenberg and Elizabeth J. Thomson

WOMEN'S HEALTH
Complexities and Differences
Edited by Sheryl Burt Ruzek, Virginia L. Olesen, and Adele E. Clarke

LOCALIZING AND GLOBALIZING REPRODUCTIVE TECHNOLOGIES
Edited by Ann R. Saetnan, Nelly Oudshoorn, and Marta Kirejczyk

LISTEN TO ME GOOD
The Life Story of an Alabama Midwife
Margaret Charles Smith and Linda Janet Holmes